The Theological Voice
of Wolf Wolfensberger

The Theological Voice of Wolf Wolfensberger has been co-published simultaneously as *Journal of Religion, Disability & Health*, Volume 4, Numbers 2/3 2001.

The *Journal of Religion, Disability & Health* Monographic "Separates"

(formerly the *Journal of Religion in Disability & Rehabilitation* series)*

For information on previous journal issues of the *Journal of Religion in Disability & Rehabilitation* series, please contact: The Haworth Press, Inc., 10 Alice Street, Binghamtom, NY 13904-1580 USA.

Below is a list of "separates," which in serials librarianship means a special issue simultaneously published as a special journal issue or double-issue *and* as a "separate" hardbound monograph. (This is a format which we also call a "DocuSerial.")

"Separates" are published because specialized libraries or professionals may wish to purchase a specific thematic issue by itself in a format which can be separately cataloged and shelved, as opposed to purchasing the journal on an on-going basis. Faculty members may also more easily consider a "separate" for classroom adoption.

"Separates" are carefully classified separately with the major book jobbers so that the journal tie-in can be noted on new book order slips to avoid duplicate purchasing.

You may wish to visit Haworth's website at . . .

http://www.HaworthPress.com

. . . to search our online catalog for complete tables of contents of these separates and related publications.

You may also call 1-800-HAWORTH (outside US/Canada: 607-722-5857), or Fax: 1-800-895-0582 (outside US/Canada: 607-771-0012), or e-mail at:

getinfo@haworthpressinc.com

The Theological Voice of Wolf Wolfensberger, edited by William C. Gaventa, MDiv, and David L. Coulter, MD (Vol. 4, No. 2/3, 2001). *This thought-provoking volume presents Wolfensberger's challenging, outrageous, and inspiring ideas on the theological significance of disabilities, including the problem with wheelchair access ramps in churches, the meaning of suffering, and the spiritual gifts of the mentally retarded.*

A Look Back: The Birth of the Americans with Disabilities Act, edited by Robert C. Anderson, MDiv (Vol. 2, No. 4, 1996).* *Takes you to the unique moment in American history when persons of many different backgrounds and with different disabilities united to press Congress for full recognition and protection of their rights as American citizens.*

Pastoral Care of the Mentally Disabled: Advancing Care of the Whole Person, edited by Sally K. Severino, MD, and Reverend Richard Liew, PhD (Vol. 1, No. 2, 1994).* *"A great book for theologians with a refreshing dogma-free approach; thought provoking for physiotherapists and all other human beings!" (The Chartered Society of Physiotherapy)*

The Theological Voice of Wolf Wolfensberger

William C. Gaventa, MDiv
David L. Coulter, MD
Editors

The Theological Voice of Wolf Wolfensberger has been co-published simultaneously as *Journal of Religion, Disability & Health*, Volume 4, Numbers 2/3 2001.

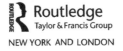

Routledge
Taylor & Francis Group

NEW YORK AND LONDON

First Published by

The Haworth Press, Inc., 10 Alice Street, Binghamton, NY 13904-1580

Transferred to Digital Printing 2008 by Routledge
270 Madison Ave, New York NY 10016
2 Park Square, Milton Park, Abingdon, Oxon, OX14 4RN

The Theological Voice of Wolf Wolfensberger has been co-published simultaneously as *Journal of Religion, Disability & Health,* Volume 4, Numbers 2/3 2001.

The development, preparation, and publication of this work has been undertaken with great care. However, the publisher, employees, editors, and agents of The Haworth Press and all imprints of The Haworth Press, Inc., including The Haworth Medical Press® and Pharmaceutical Products Press®, are not responsible for any errors contained herein or for consequences that may ensue from use of materials or information contained in this work. Opinions expressed by the author(s) are not necessarily those of The Haworth Press, Inc.

Cover design by Thomas J. Mayshock Jr.

Library of Congress Cataloging-in-Publication Data

The theological voice of Wolf Wolfensberger / William C. Gaventa, David L. Coulter, editors.
    p. cm.
    Includes bibliographical references and index.
    ISBN 0-7890-1314-2 (alk. paper) – ISBN 0-7890-1315-0 (pbk. : alk. paper)
    1. Mental retardation–Religious aspects–Christianity. 2. Church work with the mentally handicapped. 3. Wolfensberger, Wolf. I. Gaventa, William C. II. Coulter, David L. III. Journal of religion, disability & health.

BV4461 .T48 2001
261.8′322′092–dc21
                                       2001022284

Publisher's Note
The publisher has gone to great lengths to ensure the quality of this reprint but points out that some imperfections in the original may be apparent.

Indexing, Abstracting & Website/Internet Coverage

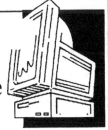

This section provides you with a list of major indexing & abstracting services. That is to say, each service began covering this periodical during the year noted in the right column. Most Websites which are listed below have indicated that they will either post, disseminate, compile, archive, cite or alert their own Website users with research-based content from this work. (This list is as current as the copyright date of this publication.)

Abstracting, Website/Indexing Coverage .... Year When Coverage Began

- *Applied Social Sciences Index & Abstracts (ASSIA)*
  (Online: ASSI via Data-Star) (CDRom: ASSIA Plus)
  <http://www.bowker-saur.co.uk> 1994

- *BUBL Information Service: An Internet-based Information*
  Service for the UK higher education community
  <URL: http://bubl.ac.uk/> 1995

- *CINAHL (Cumulative Index to Nursing & Allied Health*
  Literature), in print, also on CD-ROM from CD PLUS,
  EBSCO, and SilverPlatter, and online from CDP Online
  (formerly BRS), Data-Star, and PaperChase.
  (Support materials include Subject Heading List,
  Database Search Guide, and instructional video) 1994

- *CNPIEC Reference Guide: Chinese National Directory*
  of Foreign Periodicals 1996

- *Family Studies Database (online and CD/ROM)*
  <www.nisc.com> 1996

- *FINDEX <www.publist.com>* 1999

(continued)

- *Human Resources Abstracts (HRA)* **1994**
- *IBZ International Bibliography of Periodical Literature* **1996**
- *Occupational Therapy Index/AMED Database* **1994**
- *Orere Source, The (Pastoral Abstracts)* **1999**
- *Periodica Islamica* **1994**
- *REHABDATA <http://www.naric.com/naric>* **1999**
- *Religious & Theological Abstracts. For a free search & more information visit our website at: <http://www.rtabst.org>* . . **1999**
- *Sage Family Studies Abstracts (SFSA)* **1994**
- *Theology Digest (also made available on CD-ROM)* **1994**

Special Bibliographic Notes related to special journal issues (separates) and indexing/abstracting:

- indexing/abstracting services in this list will also cover material in any "separate" that is co-published simultaneously with Haworth's special thematic journal issue or DocuSerial. Indexing/abstracting usually covers material at the article/chapter level.

- monographic co-editions are intended for either non-subscribers or libraries which intend to purchase a second copy for their circulating collections.

- monographic co-editions are reported to all jobbers/wholesalers/approval plans. The source journal is listed as the "series" to assist the prevention of duplicate purchasing in the same manner utilized for books-in-series.

- to facilitate user/access services all indexing/abstracting services are encouraged to utilize the co-indexing entry note indicated at the bottom of the first page of each article/chapter/contribution.

- this is intended to assist a library user of any reference tool (whether print, electronic, online, or CD-ROM) to locate the monographic version if the library has purchased this version but not a subscription to the source journal.

- individual articles/chapters in any Haworth publication are also available through the Haworth Document Delivery Service (HDDS).

The Theological Voice
of Wolf Wolfensberger

CONTENTS

RESPONDERS

BOOK REVIEW

WOLF WOLFENSBERGER RESPONDS

ABOUT THE EDITORS

William C. Gaventa, MDiv, is Coordinator of Community and Congregational Supports at the Elizabeth M. Boggs Center on Developmental Disabilities, the University Affiliated Program of New Jersey. He also coordinates a training and technical assistance team for the New Jersey Self Determination Initiative, which now supports more than 125 individuals and their families. Mr. Gaventa also served as Coordinator of Family Support for the Georgia Developmental Disabilities Council, Chaplain and Coordinator of Religious Services for the Monroe Developmental Center, and Executive Secretary for the Religion Division of the AAMR since 1985. He completed a term on the Board of Directors of the AAMR, and serves on the Board of the National Federation of Interfaith Volunteer Caregivers.

David L. Coulter, MD, is Associate Professor of Pediatrics and Neurology and Director of Pediatric Neurology at Boston University School of Medicine. During a fellowship in ethics at Harvard Medical School, he worked to develop a broad-based spiritual basis for bioethics. Dr. Coulter leads a group at Boston Medical Center that explores the role of spirituality in pediatrics. His research focuses on issues faced by children with disabilities and their families who belong to various cultures. Dr. Coulter is active in the American Association on Mental Retardation and the Greater Boston Arc, and has been a consultant to the Massachusetts Department of Mental Retardation.

Preface

No one is neutral about Wolf Wolfensberger. I do not think he would allow it. Hank Bersani writes, "Wolfensberger draws controversies as a flame draws moths." He means to shake us up, challenge our assumptions and make us think. Like Dennis Schurter, I think of Wolfensberger as being like an Old Testament prophet, sure of himself, unafraid, willing to use "extreme terminology" to get our attention, but usually at least two steps ahead of the rest of us. If one listens carefully to what he has to say, one is forced to take a position either in agreement or opposition. And even if one agrees with him, he may still argue the point and keep challenging us to seek the truth.

This volume honors Wolfensberger in the way he might appreciate best, by stimulating vital discussion of some critical issues concerning religion, disability and health. This is not an empty celebratory tribute or festschrift. Rather, we have sought to provoke debate between Wolfensberger and the reader through a dialogue between him and three responders. We first reprint seven of Wolfensberger's papers which present his religious and spiritual viewpoint on disability and which are not widely available. We selected three responders to represent the readership and asked them to read and comment on Wolfensberger's papers. Dennis Schurter is a chaplain who has been active in the field of mental retardation for many years and who speaks of Wolfensberger's influence on him and the field. By contrast, Eric Pridmore is a graduate student in religion and disability for whom the encounter with Wolfensberger is new. Sandra Friedman is a leading physician in the field who encounters Wolfensberger from the dual perspective of a Jewish woman and a health care provider. We asked Kenneth Tittle, also a leading physician in the field, to review one of Wolfensberger's books which relates specifically to the intersection of religion, disability and health. Finally, we gave Professor Wolfensberger the opportunity to respond to the responders and to have the last word.

[Haworth indexing entry note]: "Preface." Coulter, David L. Published in *The Theological Voice of Wolf Wolfensberger* (ed: William C. Gaventa, and David L. Coulter) The Haworth Pastoral Press, an imprint of The Haworth Press, Inc., 2001, pp. xi-xii. Single or multiple copies of this article are available for a fee from The Haworth Document Delivery Service [1-800-342-9678, 9:00 a.m. - 5:00 p.m. (EST). E-mail address: getinfo@haworthpressinc.com].

xi

How might the reader best use this material? Let me state at the outset that I do not believe Professor Wolfensberger is always right. And I would expect him to argue with me about it. The conjunctive stage of faith development (according to James Fowler) embraces polarities and is alert to paradox and the need for multiple interpretations of reality. I suspect Wolfensberger is at that point where he expects disagreement and is perfectly comfortable with the fact that he believes what he believes and that others believe something different. Although I may disagree with some of his arguments in the articles reprinted in this volume, I have been challenged by them and appreciate the tremendous impact he has had on the development of my own beliefs. In particular, he alerted me to the very real risks of what he calls "death-making" long before the current societal interest in euthanasia and assisted suicide for people with disabilities.

Do not read these articles with the idea that you must agree with everything Professor Wolfensberger has written. Read them carefully and think about what he is saying. Take a stance either in agreement or in opposition and think about why you may agree or disagree with him. Then read his articles again and see if he can convince you or if you can argue a convincing alternative point of view. Read the responses to his articles and see if they support your arguments, and then read Wolfensberger's responses to the commentaries. Maybe he will change your mind, maybe he will not. Whatever happens, you will come away from this issue of the Journal with a stronger sense of what you believe and why you believe it. Wolfensberger concludes his "Response to the Responders" by writing, "This format of debate and analysis is very much what we need because I expect it will lead to much clarification of thought." And I think that is the best way to honor Professor Wolfensberger for the enormous impact he has had on all of us.

David L. Coulter, MD
Co-Editor

A Note of Appreciation

This book could not have happened without the cooperation and assistance of many people. That is, in fact, a testimony in itself, both to the contributions of Wolf Wolfensberger and to the crucial importance of the questions and issues which he raises in these papers.

This volume was born in a vision to "resurrect" the papers and presentations that Wolf has made over the past quarter century, primarily in two arenas, the Religion Division of the AAMR and the National Apostolate for Inclusion Ministries (NAIM, formerly the National Apostolate for Persons with Mental Retardation). Most of the presentations, except the last one, had been published in the earlier journals or publications of these two groups. We are very grateful to the Religion Division of the AAMR, and to NAIM for permission to republish these papers.

Why do so? For one, in my opinion, many of them are classics. I will never forget being present for Wolf's presentation of "An Attempt to Find an Adequate Theological Foundation." I remember reading his early version of the Prophetic "Voice and Presence" and resonating, as a young chaplain in one of the hellacious large institutions not far from Syracuse, with the words and thoughts that no one was acknowledging those days, i.e., the ways that people with mental retardation were teaching me. They are both papers I have continued to copy and give out, time and time again, to clergy and others coming into the field. One of Wolf's real contributions is the way he places his questions and issues in an historical context. Thus, from one perspective, this book is one attempt to thank him, in kind.

Thus, I "grew up" as a young chaplain with Wolf Wolfensberger as a living presence in the field. Most other contributors to this volume, i.e., Hank Bersani, David Coulter, Dennis Schurter, and Sandra Friedman, did the same. Hank Bersani was our "insider" from Syracuse. Dennis Schurter has been involved as a chaplain and with the Religion Division of the AAMR for the past twenty-five years, and currently serves as its President. We are very

[Haworth indexing entry note]: "A Note of Appreciation." Gaventa, Bill. Published in *The Theological Voice of Wolf Wolfensberger* (ed: William C. Gaventa, and David L. Coulter) The Haworth Pastoral Press, an imprint of The Haworth Press, Inc., 2001, pp. xiii-xiv. Single or multiple copies of this article are available for a fee from The Haworth Document Delivery Service [1-800-342-9678, 9:00 a.m. - 5:00 p.m. (EST). E-mail address: getinfo@haworthpressinc.com].

xiii

grateful to each of them for their wonderful pieces. Sandra Friedman took on the challenge of writing from both her professional role as a pediatrician and her Jewish tradition. Eric Pridmore and Ken Tittle came to his works with fresh perspectives, coming out of their primary involvement with issues of disability and religion in the world of physical disabilities.

It also took many hands and hours to get these papers from old formats, in some cases mimeographed journals (remember the mimeograph) and into new digitalized wineskins. Laurie Bleakley, a Lutheran seminarian and trainee at The Boggs Center-UAP in 1998-99, did much of the first work. She is now an Associate Pastor. Susan Thomas, Wolf Wolfensberger's able associate, compared new versions with older manuscripts, and worked with me till we got it right. Precision and thoroughness have long been "signs" that Wolf was involved. But we also left Wolf's unique use of English words, or invention of new ones, as they stood. My MS Word based spell-check might not like it, but the accuracy of a version faithful to the historical voice demands it.

Our hope is that from whatever perspective and historical vantage point you enter these papers and the dialogue in this work, you will be challenged, nurtured, and enriched.

Bill Gaventa, MDiv
Co-Editor

INTRODUCTION

Wolf Wolfensberger:
Scholar, Change Agent, and Iconoclast

Hank Bersani Jr., PhD

Who is Wolf Wolfensberger, and why are we devoting an entire publication to his work? Well, it occurs to us that some people are quite familiar with the "disability" side of Dr. Wolfensberger. Readers may know several of his books (Wolfensberger, 1972, 1983; Wolfensberger and Zauha, 1973) and even if they disagree with some of his positions, they are quite familiar with his position on topics such as integration, deinstitutionalization, and program evaluation. Many readers will be surprised to see that he has so many things to say in the area of religion.

On the other hand, there is no doubt readers who are familiar with Dr. Wolfensberger's teachings in the area of religion and spirituality, which while they are always in the context of people who are devalued, do not often make clear the clinical and social policy background from which he writes. Just as this volume seeks to bring together areas of spirituality, disability and health, so do the writings of Dr. Wolfensberger run the gamut from clinical, psycho-

Hank Bersani Jr. is Associate Professor of Special Education, Western Oregon University, 345 North Monmouth Avenue, Monmouth, OR 97361 (E-mail: bersanh@ wou.edu).

[Haworth co-indexing entry note]: "Wolf Wolfensberger: Scholar, Change Agent, and Iconoclast." Bersani, Hank, Jr. Co-published simultaneously in *Journal of Religion, Disability & Health* (The Haworth Pastoral Press, an imprint of The Haworth Press, Inc.) Vol. 4, No. 2/3, 2001, pp. 1-9; and: *The Theological Voice of Wolf Wolfensberger* (ed: William C. Gaventa, and David L. Coulter) The Haworth Pastoral Press, an imprint of The Haworth Press, Inc., 2001, pp. 1-9. Single or multiple copies of this article are available for a fee from The Haworth Document Delivery Service [1-800-342-9678, 9:00 a.m. - 5:00 p.m. (EST). E-mail address: getinfo@haworthpressinc.com].

1

logical issues in mental retardation, to the role of life, death, and spirituality in all of our lives, including those of us with disabilities.

The purpose of this volume is to feature some of the most challenging writings of this prolific author, who has made his mark on so many aspects of the fields addressed; people with disabilities, issues of religion and spirituality, and health issues.

I remember the day I first met Dr. Wolfensberger. I was a masters student at Syracuse University, and he had just come to join the faculty. The program was abuzz that the developer of the normalization principle was going to be on campus. He was giving his first formal address, and we all filled the room to hear–faculty and students alike. I arrived early and watched as the janitor prepared the room for the lecture with enormous attention to detail. Lining up the chairs just so, wiping down the speaker's table, checking and double-checking the overhead projector and screen. It seemed that even the janitor knew that this was the presentation of the year. Finally, dusting the lens on the projector one last time, the janitor (one I had not seen in the building before) seemed to declare the room ready. He went and stood in the far corner. In his work boots, dark brown pants and dark brown turtleneck, it appeared he was going to stay for the lecture. Burton Blatt, Director of the Division of Special Education, stepped up to the podium and read the impressive credentials of Dr. Wolfensberger. As we all listened, I scanned the front, and then the rear of the room, looking for the famous speaker. Dr. Blatt completed his remarks and the janitor–or the man I thought to be the janitor–strode to the podium and began his presentation. Ironically, much of the presentation dealt with the issue of stereotypes, and although within six months I was traveling and lecturing with him, I never told him about my assumptions made on that day.

BIOGRAPHICAL SKETCH

Wolfensberger was born in Mannheim, Germany, in 1934, lived away from home for several years during World War II, and immigrated to the U.S. as a 16-year-old. He was naturalized as a US citizen in 1956. In later life, he would recount how his value system was shaped by his early years in Europe and World War II. His formal education included a bachelor's degree in philosophy at Siena College (1955) in Memphis, Tennessee (now defunct). He went on to earn a master's degree in psychology and education (1957) from St. Louis University in Missouri, and a PhD (1962) from the George Peabody College for Teachers (which later became a part of Vanderbilt University). Within the psychology program, Peabody was offering a new program not previously offered at any other university–a specialization in mental retardation. Wolfensberger was in the first cohort to graduate with this specialization. Prior to this time, there was not enough interest in the construct of mental retardation for it to warrant an individual specialty.

In the 1950s and 60s Wolfensberger had a number of clinical experiences that shaped his view of services to people with disabilities. He was a laboratory technician for a chemical company in Tennessee, and worked as a clerk-statistician at St. Louis University. Later, he served in prestigious internships with Jack Tizard and Neil O'Connor–two international leaders in psychology at the time–in England. Later, he was the Chief Psychologist at one mental retardation institution, and Director of Research and Training at another.

His groundbreaking work in the state of Nebraska from 1963 to 1971 was based at the Nebraska Psychiatric Institute, University of Nebraska. In that capacity, he headed the Nebraska Mental Retardation Manpower Development and Training Station. He was also influential in the development of the Eastern Nebraska Community Office of Mental Retardation (ENCOR), which attracted national and international attention for over a decade. At that time, the services in ENCOR were so impressive, that leaders from across the US, Europe, and even Scandinavia came to visit and to learn about the construct of community services.

By 1971 Wolfensberger was invited to serve as a visiting scholar at the Canadian Institute on Mental Retardation located at York University (now the Roeher Institute) in Toronto where he stayed for two years with a joint appointment as special lecturer in the Department of Psychology.

In 1973, Wolfensberger joined the graduate faculty at the Syracuse University Division of Special Education and Rehabilitation where he created his Training Institute. After several moves and career changes in his early life, Syracuse has continued to be his home and his base of operations for over 25 years now.

International Recognition

Wolfensberger has been widely recognized and honored in the areas of mental retardation and psychology. He has been elevated to the status of Fellow in the American Association on Mental Deficiency (now American Association on Mental Retardation), the American Psychological Association, and the American Association for the Advancement of Science. His affiliations and memberships reflect the diversity of his interests and his thinking. He has been a member of Common Cause, the World Future Society, the American Association of University Professors; and local and national Associations for Retarded Citizens/Arc's. He is a lifetime member of Sigma Chi, and has been listed in *American Men and Women of Science*, *World Who's Who in the Midwest*, the *Dictionary of International Biography*, *Community Leaders of America*, and *Leaders in Education*.

In 1991, an article in *Education and Training in Mental Retardation* reported on a study to determine the 25 top classic works in the literature on mental retardation. Dr. Wolfensberger earned two places on the list, with his

1983 article on "Social Role Valorization" ranked as 17th, and his 1972 book on normalization ranked #1. Most recently, the American Association on Mental Retardation (AAMR) named him as one of 36 historic figures in the field.

Wolfensberger is the author of well over three hundred publications from 1957 to the present, including 27 books and monographs, 17 book chapters, over 200 articles and book reviews, and a handful of poems.

Dr. Wolfensberger is also a member of the U.S. Chess Federation, with a rating of "U.S. Chess Expert," was a co-founder of the Memphis Philatelic Society, and has been a member of various environmental groups including the Sierra Club.

Wolfensberger is married, and he and his wife Nancy have raised three grown children, each successful in their own right.

Ever the Iconoclast

Wolfensberger draws controversies as a flame draws moths. His pressure in the 1970s for us to be careful about our language shaped the discussion about people with disabilities. He, more than any other writer, speaker, and influencer of the philosophy of our field, led to the shift from talking about "children" when we clearly mean adults, and away from talking about mental age and IQ as if they were self-defining. He urged us to not take ordinary life activities and call them therapy in the context of disability or health care need. For example, enjoying gardening–for people with disabilities becoming horticulture therapy. Benefiting from having a pet becomes pet therapy, and finding riding a horse to be fun and a good source of exercise becomes equestrian therapy.

However, although he taught us to watch our language, he continues to find use for linguistic constructs that many of us have abandoned. He prefers the word "handicapped" to "disabled" citing the etymology of the prefix "dis" meaning "not able," and saying that people with handicaps may be able, but handicapped. In fact, he often prefers to refer to people who are "wounded," or "psychically wounded." He avoids so-called "People First" language, suggested by so many people with disabilities, and continues to write about "handicapped people." More importantly, the clinician in him clings to the term mental retardation as a legitimate diagnostic label even though he has railed at stereotyping and the excessive focus on diagnostics. And last but not least, he sometimes writes about Satan as a specific individual. There are few mental retardation professionals, people with disabilities, or clergy who do not take issue with some aspect of his writing.

Once writing extensively about the essential role of consumer involvement in human services, he now writes about people with cognitive disabilities as being prophets, and as vulnerable and needing protection in the medical system, but no longer addresses the issue of them also being consumers, with power, self-advocates, capable of contributing to their own well being as well as ours, and able to advocate on their own behalf, individually and corporately. He does still write about people representing themselves and speaking on their own behalf, but in a very nuanced fashion. He explains that we all need the advocacy of others at times, but that some people cannot advocate for themselves at all and will need to rely on the advocacy of others. For this reason, he prefers the term interdependence to the more popular term "self-determination" which he sees as more radical. Similarly, he also clings to the use of Negroid and Caucasoid when referring to racial differences that others call black and white, seeking greater clarity in older terms he feels is lacking in more popular formulations.

Words and Phrases

Sadly, although he writes prolifically, only limited numbers of pages have found their way into refereed journals in the last decade–an average of one journal article per year. Many of his ideas have been promulgated via monographs, books, chapters, and an extensive number of training workshops (running 3-6 days) all across the US, Canada, Australia and the UK, and self-published newsletters and training materials. Thus, the careful reader of professional (or religious) journals might have missed my favorite insight from this scholar, his point in his workshops that "human service workers lust for and fornicate with idolatrous technologies." Yet there is no more dramatic description of the attraction that fads have in our field–in our search for a cure for disability.

Wolfensberger is well known for his penchant for long titles, and "Wolfisms." As pointed out in a review of his recent book (in this volume), his most recent 80-page booklet has a title of some 24 words. His Training Institute at Syracuse University is fully titled The Training Institute for Human Service Planning, Leadership & Change Agentry. An article published in 1994 (with Susan Thomas) is titled: Constraints and cautions in formulating recommendations to a service especially in the context of an external PASS or PASSING evaluation. Students of the principle of Normalization, and the related measurement system of Program Analysis of Service Systems (PASS) will recognize terms such as "deviancy image juxtaposition," "congregation and assimilation potential," "age appropriateness," and of course "intensity of relevant programming."

In later years, the principle of normalization gave way to the construct of Social Role Valorization–in an effort to clarify some of the misinterpretations and conscious bastardizations of the earlier principle.

Day to Day Application of Philosophy

As a practicing Catholic working at a medical school in the area of "disability," I see Wolfensberger all the time. Not the person, but his work. Once familiar with his critiques, his insight, and his world view, one cannot look at things the same way ever again.

I recently spoke at Grand Rounds for our hospital obstetric and Gynecology Department. The "clinical case" being discussed was a 15-year-old female who was said to have severe mental retardation. While undergoing ovarian surgery, the family suggested, "while you are in there, just take out her whole uterus" and the surgeon agreed and scheduled the procedures. When at the last minute, the hospital patient advocate intervened and told the physician and the family that such a sterilization could not be allowed, they were outraged, and the surgeon called for a Grand Rounds session on the "case." The Grand Rounds discussion brought up so many issues that can be found in Dr. Wolfensberger's teaching. One group continually referred to the "patient," her various diagnoses, and especially the estimates of her low IQ. They focused their attention on the procedure and the medical judgment of the surgeon (not just a physician, but a surgeon!). Others in the room referred to the individual by her name, recounted her likes and dislikes, how she spends her days, (and activities that belie the diagnosis of severe mental retardation). The incident so clearly reflected the battle as sketched by Wolfensberger so many times, although one did not need to see Satan to see the conflicting world views.

Of course there were comments about the need for the surgeon to be in control. There were appeals made to the rights of the parents to determine what is best for their daughter. There were arguments that sterilization now was preferable to the likelihood and danger of pregnancy later (although she was not sexually active, and had not reached puberty). There were arguments about liability, medical malpractice insurance, and legal determinations. The surgery had been planned (plotted?) and without her knowledge or consent; without external review and on the basis of a dubious label of severe mental retardation. Most telling of all the comments to me was made by an ob-gyn resident who replied to the panel discussion about the ethical issues of sterilizing a 15-year-old. "I guess I have the advantage of not being burdened by ethical training like the rest of you." A vision of the hospital as an ethics-free zone. All I could do was to mutter to myself "What would Wolfie say if he was here now?" The issues Dr. Wolfensberger wrestles with and writes about are not intellectual discussions of angels dancing on the head of a pin. One needs only to accompany an individual with a disability into a hospital to know that he is dispensing practical, hands-on advice.

Enormous Background Effect on the Field

The concepts and constructs of Wolfensberger have become a part of our disability lexicon, so much so, that current students and authors may use terms without citing (or even knowing) their origins. As I was writing this piece, my July/August issue of *Teaching Exceptional Children* arrived. The final article in the issue is titled "Digitizing the community 'normalizes' students." Forgetting for a moment the irony of promoting technology (of which Wolfensberger is so suspicious) the term 'normalize' is regarded as so commonplace, that it is not defined, it is not even referenced, the construct of normalizing just *is*. While even Wolfensberger will acknowledge the Scandinavian roots of the concept, it is clearly he who made it a comprehensive principle in human services, and the defining principle of many of the reforms of the last 25 years.

Spiritual Radicalization

Wolfensberger's spiritual approach evolved slowly, to the point at which it overtook his more professional interests. One obvious change in Dr. Wolfensberger's work over time has been the change from a very professional, psychological research, through a period of social change and public policy, to a near total domination of the role of spirituality.

In the 1960s Wolfensberger published extensively in psychology journals, and in the scholarly forums of a researcher. Early publications in the journal *Mental Retardation,* and the *American Journal of Mental Deficiency,* include topics such as "Stimulus intensity and duration effects on EEG and GSR responses of normals and retardates" and "Age variations in Vineland SQ scores for the four levels of adaptive behavior of the 1959 AAMD behavioral classification." However, his publications quickly shifted to issues of service planning, delivery, and the devaluation and dehumanization of people based on their disabilities: "The evolution of dehumanization in our institutions" (in 1969 with W. D. White) and "An attempt to reconceptualize functions of services to the mentally retarded" (1969).

Although his writing in the 1960s was already challenging the "system," and addressed the issue of ethics, "Ethical issues in research with human subjects" (1967), there was no hint of the importance that religion and spirituality would take in the years to come. In the 60s Wolfensberger articulated problems in human service delivery, and sketched out solutions that included better measurement of quality, and funding linked to quality, better regional planning, smaller services, and a move towards getting services to see the intrinsic humanity of everyone they served.

By the 1970s, Wolfensberger had formalized two constructs that would shape the face of disability services into the next millennium; the principle of normalization; and the construct of Citizen Advocacy. Although the concept of normalization has its roots in Scandinavia, it was Wolfensberger and his 1972 publication *The principle of normalization in human services* that described the concept in a compelling manner for American readers, and formalized a lexicon and a "big picture" that became the backbone for advocacy efforts of the 70s and 80s. Simultaneously, Wolfensberger released his publication *Program Analysis of Service Systems (PASS),* which afforded advocates and willing service providers to quantify the extent to which any human service adhered to the principle of normalization as described by Wolfensberger.

Wolfensberger clearly saw the need to systemic social change, but even in the early 1970s he was formalizing the role for individual citizens acting on their own.

Also in the 1970s Wolfensberger was greatly influenced by the writings of Michel Foucault. He described Foucault's (1965) book *Madness and civilization* to be "a book of greatest profundity." In his review of the Foucault text he writes:

> . . . insights such as these can only bring a shudder of agonized recognition to perceptive observers, in disclosing the meanings of some of the practices which are still so universally prevalent in our society, and which are prevalent in the name of medicine, and health, religion, social order, and social charity.

Early signs of his religious interests can be seen in a 1961 article on what he referred to as the "free will controversy." The next appearance of his writing that reflects spiritual interests is in a 1973 article of reflections on the movement of L'Arche. In the mid-seventies, one cannot escape noticing a dramatic shift in the tone of his writing. In his own words, Wolfensberger pinpoints the event that precipitated the shift. He writes "After I read Stringfellow's compelling reasoning and documentation, I began to see the world in a whole new pattern." I believe that I was there the day this happened. We were conducting a workshop/retreat for the New Jersey Department of Institutions in 1975 or 1976. Wolfensberger had begun to include some spiritual information in his training, referring to Jean Vanier and the L'Arche movement, as well as the Catholic Worker Movement. He clearly saw a connection between spirituality and people with mental retardation. In fact, we were conducting the conference at a retreat house, and had a priest with us, Father Bill Cuddy, who was involved in the lives of men and women with mental retardation. One night (about 2:00 AM as I recall) Wolfensberger knocked on all of our doors, and summoned us to the common area. He announced he had just read "the most biblical book since the Bible." It was Stringfellow (1973).

Things have not been the same since.

REFERENCES

Kugel, R., & Wolfensberger, W. (Eds.) (1969) Changing patterns in residential services for the mentally retarded. Washington, DC: President's Committee on Mental Retardation.

Stringfellow, W. (1973) Count it all joy: Reflections on faith, doubt and temptation: An ethic for Christians and other aliens in a strange land. Waco, TX: Word Books.

White, W., & Wolfensberger, W. (1969) The evolution of dehumranization in out institutions. *Mental Retardation.* 7(3), 5-9.

Wolfensberger, W. (1972) The principle of normalization in human services. Toronto: National Institute on Mental Retardation.

Wolfensberger, W. (1983) Normalization-based guidance, education and supports for families of handicapped people. Toronto, Canada: National Institute on Mental Retardation.

Wolfensberger, W. and Zauha, H. (1973) Citizen advocacy and protective services for the impaired and handicapped. Toronto, Canada: National Institute on Mental Retardation.

THE THEOLOGICAL PAPERS
OF WOLF WOLFENSBERGER

The Prophetic Voice and Presence
of Mentally Retarded People
in the World Today

Wolf Wolfensberger, PhD

Wolf Wolfensberger was born in Mannheim, Germany, in 1934, and came to the United States at age 16. He majored in philosophy at Siena College in Memphis, received an MA in clinical psychology at St. Louis University, and a PhD in psychology at George Peabody College for Teachers where he specialized in mental retardation and minored in special education. His involvement with handicapped and devalued groups has been very diverse. He formulated the citizen advocacy scheme, contributed to the systematization of the normalization principle, developed methods for evaluating the quality of human services, and has been active in l'Arche. Recent interests include the history of human services, how Christian human services are characterized, and formulation of opposition to the rising endangerment of the lives of certain devalued groups in society. Since 1973, he has been a professor at Syracuse University, Division of Special Education and Rehabilitation.

Edited presentation given to the Religion Subdivision of the American Association of Mental Deficiency (AAMD) at the 100th National Conference, Chicago, May 1976, and to the International Federation of l'Arche, Chateauneuf, France, April 3, 1978. Published previously in shorter and different forms as "The Moral Challenge of Mentally Retarded Persons to Human Services" in *Information Service* (publication of the Religion Division of AAMD), 1977, 6(3), 6-16; and in *International Federation of l'Arche*, Springs of New Hope, 1978, 37-80.

[Haworth co-indexing entry note]: "The Prophetic Voice and Presence of Mentally Retarded People in the World Today." Wolfensberger, Wolf. Co-published simultaneously in *Journal of Religion, Disability & Health* (The Haworth Pastoral Press, an imprint of The Haworth Press, Inc.) Vol. 4, No. 2/3, 2001, pp. 11-48; and: *The Theological Voice of Wolf Wolfensberger* (ed: William C. Gaventa, and David L. Coulter) The Haworth Pastoral Press an imprint of The Haworth Press, Inc., 2001, pp. 11-48. Single or multiple copies of this article are available for a fee from The Haworth Document Delivery Service [1-800-342-9678, 9:00 a.m. 5:00 p.m. (EST). E-mail address: getinfo@haworthpressinc.com].

Introduction
Problems and Temptations Characteristic of Our Time
The Perception of the World by Non-Christians and Christians

The Prophetic Message of Mentally Retarded Persons
Mentally Retarded Persons Are Becoming Much More Public and Vis-
    ible
Retarded Persons Are Becoming Internationally Known
Non-Handicapped and Handicapped Persons Are Sharing Their Lives,
    Often Living Together
Retarded People Are Gentling Others
The Prophetic Manifestation of the Presence of God via Retarded
    People
Retarded People Speaking in Tongues
Retarded People May Withstand Their Culture
Retarded People May Be Parodying Intellectualism
The Dance of Spiritual Joy
Retarded People Are Beginning to Be Persecuted and Martyred

Implications of the Prophetic Message of the Mentally Retarded

The Bankruptcy of Intellectual and Technological Achievement
The Importance of Shared Worship with Retarded People
The Importance of Other Genuine Sharing with Retarded People
Those Allied with Severely Handicapped People Must Be Prepared to
    Be Persecuted and Martyred

A Concluding Personal Note
Appendix

INTRODUCTION

The thesis of my presentation is that mentally retarded people play a
unique prophetic role in this age. Christians who are allied with the mentally
retarded need to fully understand that role, and other Christians (especially
human service workers) should be aware of the phenomenon. In my remarks,
I will lean heavily on *An Ethic for Christians and Other Aliens in a Strange
Land* (Stringfellow, 1973).

Christians have always been called to see the world differently from non-
Christians, namely, to perceive the world more in the light of God's word,
revelation, and intent; and perhaps in a sense, to perceive the world a little
more the way God might perceive it. Prophets and saints have done this
traditionally–but always at a high cost. If they perceived the hidden absurdities

of their age, and then interpreted these absurdities as absurdities, they were ridiculed for their apparently far-fetched interpretations; and if these interpretations threatened the powerful, the interpreters were frequently persecuted. Indeed, tradition has it that just about every prophet of the Old Testament was martyred. We do not have historical documentation, but Christ himself, as well as the Apostles, repeatedly spoke of this as a fact to their contemporaries.

If we take a long perspective of history, it seems that each era not only recapitulates the same human fall, weaknesses and offenses, but that in addition, Satan manages to present ever new and even unique patterns of problems and temptations, which in turn result in patterns of sins that may also be more specific to that age. For instance, a recurring temptation to, and offense of, the early Jews was idolatry and worship of graven images believed to be God. During the Roman Empire, a characteristic pattern was the deification of Caesar. In the medieval age, an almost universal pattern was the glorification of violence, even by the Church. The Church even justified Christians going to war against Christians. In the light of modern times, slavery (until the mid-1800s) may have been a special patterned evil. Every era was so wrapped up in itself that it was always difficult, even for the faithful, to discern the signs of the time. Therefore, we can ask a provocative question: what might be the specific or even unique problem patterns and temptations of our own age now.

PROBLEMS AND TEMPTATIONS
CHARACTERISTIC OF OUR TIME

The one thing that is certainly unique, whatever else there may be about this age, is the deification of a "successful" technology; and technology has achieved a power that, without doubt, is unique in history. This technological power can not only put people on the moon but, for the first time in human history, it can eradicate all human life. This situation is very different from all other ages. There always existed the potential to conduct warfare, but there never existed the potential to eradicate all human life. Contrary to what most people think, this eradication can be achieved not only through nuclear warfare, but through at least five other means, such as bacterial warfare, genetic engineering and accidents, atmospheric and climatic changes and manipulations, etc.

Aside from potential total destruction, it is the very technology at its height that is now creating, or has already created, a non-functional earth which is about to collapse under the weight of the complexity of technology and of its products, such as overpopulation and (what is often overlooked by contemporary people) an unmanageably huge and complex social, political, mechanical and industrial system. The systems we are creating escape the human capability of management.

In the last few years, I have become vastly more sensitized to the messages that are contained in events, occurrences, and phenomena. I no longer see, hear, and read many things merely on the level at which they occur. For example, we all hear a lot of fire engines and police sirens going by; as I sit in my office on the university hill in Syracuse, I hear the sirens go by three and four times a day, and often I hear them at home at night. On the one hand, you may just hear sirens. On the other hand, what does it tell you when sirens scream by four times a day?

One day I asked myself, "Is there a message in all this siren noise?" and I began to no longer hear sirens. I was beginning to hear something being said–or more properly, being screamed. What are sirens, what do they mean, why are they going by? Well, it usually means that there is trouble, there are ambulances going to accidents or even merely pretending to be on important business; there are fires or fire alarms; there are police going to emergencies; and so on. When you have sirens going by an awful lot, it means there are an awful lot of problems. In different societies at different times, there are different numbers and types of problems. When you get too many sirens, maybe there is something wrong with the society. So instead of sirens, I began to hear societal screams; it was as if society was a person screaming out. Thus, when I hear the sirens now, it is no longer a siren to me, but a message–and a potentially ominous one.

But there are so many more messages, symbols, communications. Yet we are a rather literal and prosaic society, and we do not use imagery and symbolism to the degree that some other societies do (although we do more than some others), and we often fail to read the hidden messages that may be contained in various phenomena.

THE PERCEPTION OF THE WORLD
BY NON-CHRISTIANS AND CHRISTIANS

The nonfunctionalities of our highly developed societies are a puzzling paradox to non-Christians–at least the westernized ones. We have created a "techno-god" that is expected to bring "techno-salvation." And surely, the fact that this techno-god is eating its faithful must be, or is, perceived by non-Christians as, a temporary malfunction. The non-Christian hardly has other explanations; there must be a temporary mistake that can be fixed with a little more engineering, or what in computer-language is called "de-bugging." But to the Christians who relate to the totality of the Bible and of human history, there is no paradox. Quite to the contrary; the human race, as a whole, is only marching where it has always marched–the direction has never changed, only the flags, the clothes, the shoes, the music, the language. The only new thing in the history of mankind is that during the last two thousand years, God has given a few humans the option to march to a different drummer.

At any rate, Biblically-based Christians are apt to perceive, at least in a vague sense, that our age has its version of the tower of Babel; and God is about to confound the human intellectual arrogance that tends to replace Him with science and with reason. Therefore, a Biblically-based Christian would also fully expect the presence of prophetic messages of warning about these things, because much as there seem to be distinct dysfunctionalities and problems in different eras, so each era seems to receive its special form of prophecy which is addressed uniquely to that culture, society, people, time, and needs. The prophecy has an uncanny way of fitting the problem, in terms of the imagery in the messages involved, and in terms of the level of urgency. I remember once lamenting to Jean Vanier about the incredible amount and degree of corruption and evil that exists in New York State and New York City. To me, living in the state of New York is like living at the foot of the throne of Satan: there is corruption from the top to the bottom, at every level of government, all over the state. Yet Vanier reminded me that St. Paul (Romans 5:20) said that wherever evil abounds, grace super-abounds. It is similar with prophecy. Where there is a period of particular problematicness, there we will probably also find a particularly intense level of prophecy.

Prophecy can be a very private thing, and private prophecy is probably both much more common as well as diversified than public prophecy. But I am talking now primarily about public prophecy, i.e., prophecy which is as public as are the problems, and as public as are the patterns of evil and corruption to which it is addressed. It is the public pattern of prophecy that I see as being on the same level, intensity, imagery and so on as the evil, because (and of course, it makes sense) it is this kind of prophecy that is also intended to carry its message as publicly, or at least as nearly publicly, as the message of corruption, dysfunctionality, or collapse of a particular age. It also appears that such public prophecy becomes manifest in the presence of individuals, groups or movements that are very closely tied to the Spirit. All this is fully to be expected, since God has always done these things since Biblical times, and has always sent the warnings that fit the times.

I have to admit that until about 1972, I did not believe that our age was possessed of extraordinary malfunctionalities. Then increasingly, I began to read the signs differently, to the point where I now believe we are at the point where our society is in collapse. Beginning to see things in this way, and trying to read more clearly and consciously the dysfunctionalities of our age, it occurred to me that one way to understand them better is by (oddly enough) using the scientific principle of "obverting." In science, when you have a statement that expresses some scientific relationship (e.g., X causes Y), sometimes you can reverse the directionality of the statement, giving you a new and revealing way of looking at the relationships implied (e.g., if Y can be observed to be present, is X operative?). So instead of asking "Where or what are the dysfunctionalities?", one way of discerning dysfunctionalities is to ask "Where or what are the prophecies?", because if you can identify the prophecy, its form, its messenger, and its message, then that will likely tell you what the problem is.

So I asked myself, what are the prophetic signs which appear to be unique or very special to our day, which are very different from what they have been at other times? By asking, I did not mean to deny that routine and especially private prophecy does not continue; ordinary, run-of-the-mill prophecy seems to be an ongoing phenomenon. But in addition, what are the forms of prophecy which appear to be different in our age than in other ages? Where and how is the Spirit active today in a way that is different from the way it may have been in other eras?

As I posed these questions to myself over the past few years, I began to read both the signs of dysfunctionality and of prophecy in a different and clearer fashion, and I read one very, very powerful prophetic message, coming from mentally retarded people. For instance, I considered that it should not be unexpected if divine messages about the present patterning of offenses should come from people who, in their roles and identities, are exactly the opposite of what our era idolatrates. So who and what is the opposite?

The opposite is a person who is not intellectual, not scientific, not technological, and not academic; who does simple instead of complex things; who cannot cope with complexity and technology which passes him by; and who, possibly, is despised for lack of modernity and intellectuality. Is that not the retarded person of our age?

But if it is, is there any evidence that God has thrust retarded people into a prophetic role? I submit to you that there is indeed, and that there are at least ten such signs.

THE PROPHETIC MESSAGE
OF MENTALLY RETARDED PERSONS

Mentally Retarded Persons Are Becoming
Much More Public and Visible

There are a number of remarkable things going on in our age that involve and affect mentally retarded people. One of these, though remarkable, would not mean anything by itself if it were not part of a pattern, namely, the remarkable high public visibility of retarded people. That, of course, could just be an interesting secular coincidence, but nevertheless, let us start off with that. Mentally retarded people are now visible; you can see them everywhere. Sometimes, their visibility may be a tragic one, in that we may see the people who have been dumped from the institutions walking the streets, and we can recognize them on sight as being retarded because of the way they are neglected, by their acultural appearance, their odd behaviors, and so on. We may also hear more about abuses committed on retarded people in the community, of which more is said later. On the other hand, we are also seeing more retarded persons in constructive contexts, for example, at conventions. In our field, you formerly never saw retarded people coming to meetings and conventions, but now it is rather routine; and at a lot of both general public as well as professional and parent group events, you do see retarded people where formerly there were none. There is nothing remarkable anymore in seeing retarded people in industry, schools, churches, group homes and neighborhoods, streets, shops, on the city buses, and so on.

So all of these retarded people then become a reminder, through their visibility, of the opposite of the techno-god. The very fact that retarded people, even more than non-retarded people, in many ways look alike is remarkable. To me it is almost like the medieval cathedral–pardon the analogy–from which the gargoyles have been looking down into the marketplace for hundreds and hundreds of years, as if to say: I am always there, looking at the hustle and the bustle and the business. The recurring familiar appearance of so many retarded people seems to tell me that wherever I may go, there I also find the opposite of mental retardation, and especially so complexity. I may walk on the main street of Heidelberg, and there on a corner to a dark sideline stands a retarded man whom I immediately recognize, and he stands simply in the middle of the stream of the loud noises of technology, and conveys the message: I will always be here–unless you slay me. Unless you slay me, I will be here to remind you.

That one can go across the world and encounter so many retarded people who bear an uncanny resemblance to each other might be explained by showing how certain causative factors create distinct syndromes, such as Down's syndrome, which affect specified structures of the body in a similar manner, and which therefore result in a resemblance among many of the afflicted individuals. One can further argue that common patterns of experiential deprivation may result in similar bodily expressions. Even granted these arguments, there is something that touches one deeply when one encounters an individual to whom one can say mentally: "I know you. I have seen you many times before, among many peoples and races. You were here–long before I was–and you will probably still be here in your innocent simplicity and dependency when everything else has changed and perhaps gone into a frenzy of chaotic complexity." It is also moving to consider that unlike with some disorders, it is virtually certain that there will always be retarded people unless all fetuses at risk were aborted, and all infants and children who appear to have retarded mental development were put to death.

Thus, I choose to believe that the timeless archetypes of retarded persons are not merely biological accidents, and that the technical answer is one of those that may have been intended to confound the wise. The recurring bodily defects may have resulted from the laws of nature, but their timeless presence, I believe, is by divine design. The design, I believe, is not even that proposed by some people, i.e., to send mankind needy individuals to offer others an opportunity to practice charity on them and thereby earn salvation. I believe the design is more likely intended to confront human beings endlessly with themselves and their own nature and essence. Yes, the retarded person, no matter how profoundly impaired, is another version of myself and asks me questions: who am I, what am I, what am I made of, what about me is important, what is the meaning of the differences among us, how do we all fit together in society?

The reality that the retarded person is a version of myself is one from which so much can be learned and gained, and yet it is a reality which most people deny, and try to escape from. Should society really progress to the point where it willfully destroys the archetypal mentally retarded, then I think that that would be yet another sign of the advent of the end of times, because something would be destroyed that has always been an integral part of mankind, and thereby, the destruction of mankind itself must be in the works.

Retarded People Are Becoming Internationally Known

The second provocative phenomenon is an enlargement of the first one, and is nearly unique: mentally retarded people are achieving world-wide importance, and as far as I can determine, this has occurred at most once before in the history of the world (see appendix to this paper). You may wonder what I am talking about: where, who, what, how.

At least one way in which retarded people have unequivocally gained international visibility is in and through the l'Arche movement, which is a network of spiritually-oriented communities started in 1964 in France by Jean Vanier. There are now nearly 100 such residential communities all over the world, in almost every continent, with yet more in the making. In these settings (usually houses), handicapped and non-handicapped people are living together as much as possible as peers. In addition, there exist many local circles of people unified in the ideals of the l'Arche movement, either trying to open houses as focal points, or otherwise meeting in fellowship with handicapped (primarily mentally retarded) people. That movement has created world-wide community like no other movement that I know of. To begin with, there have been very few movements of international scope (Camphill being one) where mentally handicapped people were involved, and probably none where retarded people as specific individuals and not just in general were widely known by people in other member communities across the world. Further, I am not aware of any of the few international movements involving mentally handicapped people developing with such speed. In fact, in most other handicap areas, nothing of the sort seems to have happened before.

Among l'Arche groups, there is a constant interchange. People are traveling from one place to another, and so you have very intimate world-wide communion all the time. People may come halfway across the world to visit another community, become acquainted, experience fellowship, and then continue their relationships across time and distance. Unlike in some of the other world-wide movements where non-handicapped workers are the major participants, in l'Arche, the handicapped people also travel. When l'Arche people make movies or slides of some of their events, no matter where among their communities such pictures are shown, there will typically be shouts in the audience, "Hey look, there's Anne, there's George!", etc. Retarded people are important! A specific severely retarded person may be important to people halfway across the world who are not related to him or her!

Along the same lines of significance is that at least four mentally retarded individuals have written books (Hunt, 1967; De Vries-Kruit, 1971; Deacon, 1976; and Kerr, undated but apparently mid-1970s). Of these, two (Hunt, Deacon) have become well-known around the globe. Most remarkable of these four, from many standpoints, is Deacon's *Tongue Tied*. Joey Deacon had lived in a mental retardation institution in England for 42 years. He was 50 years old, with cerebral palsy, unable to care for himself in hardly any way. Someone had suggested to him once that he write his autobiography, and he thought about that idea for 12 years. He had to work out a system, because his speech was so poor that only his friend Ernie could understand. Ernie, however, could neither read nor write. Mike, though, who was another of his mates, could write ever so slowly and laboriously. So the team began, with Ernie closely watching Joey's face to get the words, then repeating them to Mike who slowly wrote them down. But the text had to be typed, so Tom, a third friend, was called in. He couldn't read or write either, but he said he would try to type the letters (with one finger) if they were spelled out to him. The group worked for 14 months to produce Joey's story, averaging 4 to 6 lines a day.

Another person who must be considered to be mentally retarded and who has achieved world-wide publicity is Shyoichiro Yamamura who was born in 1932, and who eventually developed drawing and painting skill. He specialized in the drawing of insects, frogs, and similar animals, and unlike the paintings of retarded persons that one sometimes sees on Christmas cards sold on behalf of the mentally retarded, his paintings are indeed striking in their boldness and pleasing form. His works have been exhibited in a number of art shows in Japan, and at New York University. Unfortunately, many of the books and other publications about him have not been translated from the Japanese, but Morishima has compiled a great deal of material on him in English (e.g., 1977).

One other example of the importance of retarded individuals was the impassioned public testimony of a man who had been in an institution most of his life that finally moved the plenary business meeting of the National Association for Retarded Children in 1973 to change its name from "Children" to "Citizens." Truly, 100, 50, 20, even 10 years earlier, that would have been considered so unthinkable that it would have been viewed as a miracle–but that has always been the trouble with miracles: they rarely happen at the "right" time and place; i.e., they tend to take us by surprise, and often occur in ways quite different than the ones we had thought of or prayed for. I fully expect more of these types of phenomena.

Non-Handicapped and Handicapped Persons Are Sharing Their Lives, Often Living Together

More people are deliberately and for positive reasons choosing to live with retarded persons. By and large, the pattern of the past has been that if a family had a retarded child, that family might live with its retarded child. While death rates in the general population were still high, relatives often took in the children if parents died; and once in a while, a retarded child might have been taken in by a friendly neighbor to be raised. But aside from that, the historically traditional pattern has not been one of other people choosing to share their lives with retarded people by living together.

Today, we not only see people who are willing to share their homes, but we see other forms of genuine sharing as well. I am not talking about the old commercial foster home placement and so on, but about people living together in group homes, or in so-called intentional communities, some of which can hardly be called group homes. I knew of one little residential community where there were maybe a dozen people at a time, of whom maybe half or even fewer were retarded. The group was not incorporated, there was no public funding, they merely lived together and shared. Whoever held a job put their money in the pot, and whoever needed food and shelter was provided for by whoever brought in some earnings.

Of course, more frequently, we see the sharing of the more formal group homes where non-retarded people in unprecedented number are now living with retarded people. There is more of a clear-cut staff-client definition, but it is still often gladly done, with high commitment and ideology. In addition, we see many young people who may be called assistants or relief staff, but who often have come because they want to do this kind of thing, and not so much because they are getting paid.

Aside from living together, we see much more sharing in other ways as well: going together to parties, enjoyment and recreation, worship and so on. That is what I call genuine life-sharing, to a degree that exceeds any we have known. We can think here especially of the tens of thousands of youths, some still children, in the various youth movements in mental retardation: the

Youth Associations with the Mentally Retarded in Canada, the youth group of the National Association for Retarded Citizens in the United States, and so on. Not only are there tens of thousands of them, but they do more radical, more genuine, sharing of life than most of the adult structures.

When I came into the field of mental retardation in 1957, almost everyone considered such work and commitment futile, hopeless, unrewarding, and wasted, and there were few workers in the field other than institution keepers. Today, as a university professor, I review perhaps a hundred applications for our graduate mental retardation training program every year, mostly by young people, many of whom practically beg us to enable them to live out a passionate desire to work with the retarded. We turn down about as many as we vote to admit. *O quae mutatio rerum.*

We can almost say that for the first time in the history of the world, a significant number of non-retarded people are relying on retarded people for their identity, their calling, their salvation in a sense, because it is by sharing with retarded people, and by beginning to identify with their frailty, that meaning is given to their lives. Apparently, such meaning is derived quite differently from the way in which religious orders have traditionally involved themselves in human service, because the orders have always had other options, and many of them served but did not share. But now, we have non-retarded people who, in a sense, do not see themselves as having other options. If they did not have the opportunity of sharing and even living with retarded people, they would not know what to do; they might be "lost souls," like so many people today. They really are dependent on sharing with retarded people for meaning in their lives. I find that very remarkable, and new, and moving. What does it mean? What is the message?

Retarded Persons Are Gentling Others

Fourthly, through increased social integration, retarded people are gentling a lot of non-retarded people. The presence of a retarded person is making a lot of non-retarded people more tender, nurturing affection, bring forth naturalness, and so on. I will recite a little vignette of an event where I sensed that strikingly. I was visiting a high school that included one class of severely retarded youngsters of high school age. When I approached this school, I saw numerous young people out on the parking lot smoking pot and sexing it up in the adjacent woods. Many of them looked like they had all sorts of problems, like in so many of our typical North American high schools–and which is one of the many symptoms of the collapse of our culture: children "dissolving," no longer being able to be in control of their lives, no self-control or direction, lots of drugs and sex and hedonism. That is what it looked like, with an expectancy for vandalism, and a policeman with a gun at the school door. That you have to have armed guards to control (protect?) school children rather generally all over North America is one of the many reasons why I think the system is coming apart.

At any rate, at this typically problem-ridden tough school, they had instituted a teaching pattern where they called on the non-handicapped high school youngsters to volunteer their free class periods to work on a one-to-one basis with their severely retarded age peers. At the beginning of a class period, 5 or 6 non-retarded youngsters, who are not distinguishable in appearance from the ones who are doing dubious things in the yard, come into the classroom of the severely retarded pupils in order to work on a one-to-one basis with a person who may be unattractive, odd, does not talk too well, and so on. They keep coming, week after week, for maybe a year, and even give up their free hour when they could be in the library, playing games, making out in the parking lot or the woods, or whatever.

One of the volunteers who came in as I was observing was one of the school's champion athletes. He was a big young man, all muscle, wearing a short-armed tight T-shirt despite the chilliness of that day, showing his muscles bulging because he wanted to let everyone know how strong he was. I suspect that he was one of the most glamorous, valued students in the high school, and probably a hero to the girls. He had volunteered to work with one of the severely retarded young women.

Of course, even on the merely technical and secular level, our blindness and stupidity about pedagogy is unbelievable. A teacher can try to feed stuff into youngsters' minds for years, but there is absolutely nothing like a valued age peer saying, "Hey, let's do this together." It is infinitely more powerful, revealing one of the inherent non-functionalities of segregation.

So it is no surprise that the young woman adored her volunteer tutor as if he was the big brother. Many of the girls in school would probably have loved it if he would pay attention to them, but here he was coming and working with her in his free hour. When it was time for the young man to leave, she looked up to him with a face radiant with adulation that expressed that she would do anything for him–to hell with the teacher, but anything for him. She patted him ever so lightly and said, "When are you coming back?" And the young man was visibly melting, trying to be strong, nonchalant and tough, but not quite managing it. He was being gentled under the hands of the severely retarded, rather unattractive young woman who adored him, patted him, and wanted him to come back. I would imagine it quite conceivable that experiences such as this might change the outlook on life of a young man who might otherwise be oriented toward the body, physical accomplishment, power, brute strength, and so on. By having a relationship with a weak woman who is very dependent and loves him, he no longer has to show all of this sort of bravado. That is just one little but striking example of the kind of gentling of which we are seeing a great deal. Of course, we could see even more of it if we were consciously oriented to it, and if we would only create the conditions and circumstances where this kind of thing would be more likely to take place.

In a river accident in Omaha (Nebraska) in July of 1972, when community services there were getting under way, five retarded men from one of the group homes were drowned, together with their counselor who had been one of my students. Several of the men died only because they were trying to help each other. The funeral services were strung out one after the other, as the bodies were found. For each service, each church (of several denominations) was packed full. I am not aware of this ever happening before in the history of the world, except perhaps in small village communities that have small churches, when people came because that was the thing to do. But when these people passed away who were of no visible importance, who held no public office, who, in fact, may not even have held work that was too meaningful or too real other than perhaps subsidized workshop-type positions, people who had no accomplishments in the arts or a creative field, people who did not even have attractive appearances or admired bodies–the citizens of the urban society of Omaha came to fill the churches as an affirmation that these individuals who had been taken away had brought gentleness and other precious gifts to them. In a sense, they came to witness that the deaths of these men had revealed the violence of others, because if violence had not been done, the special agency helping-form itself would probably not have been necessary. They came to witness that some people no longer believe in the supremacy of the secular worth that we are so totally wrapped up in. I am told–and it is one of my recurring regrets that I was not there–that at one of the services, a bird came flying into the church, lighted on the altar, and started singing. Of course, as we say, that was "just a coincidence."

A very similar event recently came to my attention (*Down's Syndrome News*, Feb. 1977), where 175 residents of the small town of Windsor, Missouri, came to the funeral of a 48-year old man with Down's Syndrome who had lived mostly in a local rest home, and whose whole possessions were in a shoebox when he died: a harmonica, an ashtray, toy deputy badges, a billfold full of pictures of town children with whom he had had a cordial relationship, and an old court notice that certified him as "mentally deficient."

We must remember that gentling will not happen where retarded people are segregated, because then, there is no contact through which gentling can take place.

The Prophetic Manifestation of the Presence of God via Retarded People

It is in the presence of mentally retarded people, and/or during events in which they play an important role, that the presence of God may be made powerfully manifest. We should not forget that it is quite possible for devout people never to feel a certain special overpowering sense that God is almost tangibly present in an assembly. This special presence is well known to many people in l'Arche who take it for granted, and forget that devout people can go through life and never have experienced it. So, when it does happen, one may not grasp its special meaning. One of the meanings is that "I, the Lord, cherish especially my littlest ones, the least and last from among you. It is because of them that I manifest myself now; thereby, they become the first." The Lord's presence is clear on other occasions as well, of course, but it is apparently vastly more likely to be made manifest where retarded people are worshipfully present.

I have been professionally involved with mentally retarded persons since 1955, and full-time in the field of mental retardation since 1957. But even in retrospect, it is only in the last few years that I have witnessed (or become aware of) the prophetic phenomena involving the mentally retarded. For example, it is only in the last few years that I have been having experiences such as moments of spiritual sharing and worship by groups that may be as large as over a hundred people of whom maybe half are severely retarded and otherwise handicapped, and where there may occur striking totality and pro-fundity of silence of a type which overpoweringly conveys THE PRESENCE OF GOD. I was stunned the first time I experienced this. I do not remember ever before having said or experienced THE PRESENCE OF GOD with such totality or conviction, until one such moment with a l'Arche group of re-tarded and non-retarded people. It happened in the context of a meeting involving spiritual sharing among many non-handicapped and severely–even very severely–handicapped people. In a secular context, with persons of the same degree of handicap, we may find poorly controlled behavior, talking, perhaps shouting if the event is exciting, perhaps groaning and moaning and screams, or other inappropriate behaviors, and we would say, "They're se-verely retarded, profoundly retarded, handicapped, what do you expect?"

Another time, at a l'Arche retreat attended by both retarded and non-re-tarded people, there was a man who I would expect to score in the (lower?) severely retarded range of functioning on an intelligence test. He had been in institutions all of his life, had very little speech, was epileptic, and had a very unexpressive face. But he sat all day with everyone else and prayed silently. Suddenly, about halfway through the day of prayer, he looked up, and though I usually do not understand much of what he says, he said the only loud thing he said all day. Again, I almost fell off whatever it was I was sitting on when he said slowly, loudly and clearly, "This is my body." This type of phenome-non is very similar to the one of "tongues" I will cover next.

Retarded People Speaking in Tongues

The Pentecostal story refers to a speaking in tongues where everyone can understand what the speaker is trying to say in one language even though the listeners are of different languages. In Pentecostal religious services, the phenomenon is usually different: even though the speaker and the listeners usually share the same language, the speaker is apt to speak in an ad hoc "non-language," i.e., in a language that is not used by any people. Presumably, the listeners hear the presence of the Spirit in the person's speaking. But I wonder if "speaking in tongues" does not have different or, at least, additional meanings. Maybe another form of "tongues" is (a) when a person who cannot speak, or who ordinarily does not speak, suddenly speaks or otherwise reveals important truths; (b) when a person who ordinarily speaks confusedly or unimportantly suddenly speaks clearly and "with authority" about religious and moral matters; (c) when a person with a speech impediment speaks clearly about the above matters; or (d) when religious truths, sentiments, or manifestations are being communicated or even mediated by persons who extensively or even exclusively use non-verbal, and possibly unorthodox, symbols and expressions, and/or universal symbolisms.[1]

In fact, what may have been the original intended meaning of "speaking in tongues" suggested itself to me through yet another event involving the mentally retarded. A l'Arche group of retarded and non-retarded people who could speak no Polish were making a pilgrimage to Poland. They wanted to share their joy and spiritual exuberance with the local people, but how do you do that, and let them know of the brother/sisterhood with them that you experience? The group came up with little signs such as snapping their fingers above their heads while singing simple universal phrases such as "la-la-la" and "alleluia"–and sure enough, the message came across loud and clear. People understood what they were saying. That is indeed "tongues," though different from the way we usually think of it.

Another example of tongues occurred at a fiesta which Vanier was leading, where several hundred people were together. Typically, fiestas have both their loud and their quiet moments. Often, there is singing and joyful dancing, but also moments of reflection and prayer. At one point, everyone was sitting around candles on the floor, and as Vanier was leading the reflection, the question came up: What does it mean to care for people, to love someone? A retarded man spoke up and said: "You pray together . . . stay together." Quickly, the theme transferred to "peace," and a retarded man who tends to ramble, and who spoke rather incoherently, dropped out of his ramblings the phrases: ". . . peace is the glory of God the Father . . . peace is a strong word . . . peace is the strongest thing in the world . . ." I did not trust my ears but I had heard it all clear as a bell, perfectly cohesive statements in perfect English dropping out of a background of babble. It was thrilling. He went on, and just as I was pulling myself back together, he said ". . . peace is countries together . . . holds religions together . . ." My mind reeled. A philosopher king could not have put it any better. When Vanier asked a girl who appeared to be shy and retarded what "peace" meant, she said, "I just feel like singing, make me a channel"–and everyone almost by reflex broke into the Song of St. Francis, "Make Me a Channel of Your Peace."

To conclude the discussion of tongues, I am quite prepared to accept that a believer may be moved by the Spirit to break into a "non-language" tongue as I have defined it above. However, especially in light of St. Paul's (I Corinthians 14) extensive cautions about what must have been misuse of tongues-speaking, and his distinction between tongues and prophecy, I prefer to conclude at least tentatively that the speaking in tongues that is prophetic rather than prayerful is more apt to be one of the other of tongues described above, rather than a "non-language" tongue. Is it really inconceivable that the speaking in tongues at Pentecost (Acts 2) consisted of a Spirit-filled transmission of the presence of God, His glorification, noble emotions, joy, etc., that was the universal message understood by all those present? Would it not be a glorious and significant miracle that it is only in this age and with the help of retarded people that we might have come to understand how the speaking of tongues at the first Pentecost might have taken place?

Retarded People May Withstand Their Culture

A friend (Paul Racourt) pointed out that another prophetic sign may be the fact that in the midst of the complexities and temptations of technologies and wealth, many retarded people remain remarkably untouched by the power of the mass media, and also maintain a remarkably pure simplicity and morality. That these virtues are not merely due to mental limitation is borne out by the fact that many other retarded people fall ready victim to the same things as the other people of our age.

A small but poignant contrast between the abysmal stupidity of the masses of gifted people and the simple purity of the retarded person struck me powerfully when I read a 1976 newsletter for and of employees of a state institution for the retarded (in a state where they are trying to convert all the state mental institutions into prisons). I counted over 40 stupidities, absurdities, atrocities, immoralities, self-deceptions, other-deceptions, and deviancy enlargements of retarded people in this one little issue–and then there was one letter published in it by a former resident who had been transferred to a nursing home, and the letter was a pure loving Christian sermon, theologically sound, an affirmation of the faith without deception. It could have been a credo for the employees–so many of whom seemed caught up in a systematic devaluation of their charges, and in deceiving themselves and the world.

Retarded People May Be Parodying Intellectualism

Another friend (Doug Mouncey) pointed out that many of the behaviors emitted by retarded people irritate and aggravate bright people, and that some of these behaviors may constitute a parodying of some of the intellectualisms of a culture that elevates intellect and secular achievement to an extreme. Such parodying would not be malicious, but an innocent acting out of God's derision, so to speak, at our efforts to build intellectual towers of Babel.

An example of the above might well be the behavior of a very gentle, severely retarded man who has a habit of holding a book as if he were reading in it, and then speaking very seriously as if he were reading–even though he cannot read. What makes this vignette more noteworthy than others along the same line is that the people around him are under the impression that well above 50% of the time, he is holding the book upside down.

Once we become alert to the possibility that such parodying might occur, we may perceive more of it. It certainly would be consistent with the other prophetic signs reported here. We should be especially alert to behaviors that simultaneously make no sense, are harmless, and yet vex us (using the term "us" very deliberately).

The Dance of Spiritual Joy

The dance of spiritual joy! For instance, we read about King David dancing "with all his might" before the Ark (2 Kings 6). His wife Michol could not understand it, "despised him" for it, and gave him hell. Only at fiestas with retarded participants have I seen this type of dancing–not the sexualized dancing of our age, but the dancing of love, fellowship, and the Spirit.[2] Once, in the middle of the floor, a severely retarded man who had very little speech suddenly knelt down, folded his hands and began to pray silently in total ecstatic absorption. As the other people perceived this, they joyfully began to dance around him in a circle. This was the second time that I knew THE PRESENCE OF GOD in a way I had not previously felt.

At the l'Arche pilgrimage to Canterbury Cathedral, suddenly during the Easter celebration, the retarded and non-retarded people started dancing in the aisles and before the altar. Apparently never in the history of Canterbury Cathedral had there been dancing in the sign of joy before the altar. The Dean of the Cathedral was so deeply moved that he cried. The Archbishop of Canterbury himself was so inspired by the joy of the celebration that involved so many retarded people, that in the greatest and most solemn cathedral in Britain, on the greatest and most solemn feast day of the Christian year, he rang a bell much as the Pilgrims to Canterbury traditionally have done (Shearer, 1974).

Retarded People Are Beginning to Be Persecuted and Martyred

It is both a tragic and joyful sign that a whole new wave of persecution of retarded people has broken out. Many people are not yet aware of this persecution because it is still partially hidden, but it is undoubtedly present.

Elsewhere, I am documenting the overpowering presence of all sorts of dynamics in support of legalized mass destruction of severely handicapped persons. And why should we be surprised? In the scheme of the never-ending struggle between good and evil, darkness and light, and the calling of the life on this earth versus the next, it is fully to be expected that precisely at the moment at which mentally retarded people would begin to prophesy publicly and visibly on a large scale, they would begin to be persecuted and even put to death. The logic is compelling: the world has always tried to put to death God's prophecy, and it is in the nature of God's will that prophets must be prepared to be martyrs, and disproportionately they are. The moment retarded people in significant numbers become bearers of the word of God, the principalities and powers will converge upon them to fight and stifle that form of prophecy that is so specially powerful all because of its much more miraculous nature, and because in some ways, it goes beyond what any other type of prophecy has said before. Past prophecy has said Jewish people will be destroyed, you will be going into exile, the Egyptians will beat hell out of you, and stuff like that. But these were all reversible things–in a sense, temporary things. But we have never been told in systematic prophecy that human intellect is universally bankrupt, and that millennia of technological development are at an end.

Actually, the persecution and slaughter of the retarded has already begun and is well underway. One only needs to "read" the news in a biblical rather than merely secular way. For example, I suspect that hundreds of thousands of unborn children with handicaps have been aborted; it is one form of genocide. Euthanasia is already being committed on a vast number of handicapped newborns. Euthanasia is being committed on many retarded people of all ages when quite ordinary medical supports are withheld whenever they are sick. In North America, it is dangerous for moderately or severely handicapped people to be sent to a general hospital without a friend standing watch at their bedside. Legions of retarded people are being socialized into death in nursing homes and similar facilities. In one huge nursing home in the United States, 1000 out of 2100 residents have been dying every year for several years, most of them old and/or handicapped.

Also, while in former days, there was plenty of abuse and dehumanization of residents in hospitals, nursing homes, and institutions, we are now seeing what appears to be an entirely new form and expression of abuse (which we should expect if, indeed, retarded people are assuming a new prophetic role), namely, symbolic abuse, and abuse by sound and well-heeled people.

Formerly, abuse derived overwhelmingly from three sources: (a) Under-staffing on the primary worker level, which was usually (not always!) a result of underfunding, (b) The actions of psychopathic or even sadistic individual staff members, typically on the primary worker level where personal abuse was easiest to perpetrate. Such individuals had slipped through the personnel screening and were usually discharged when found out, and (c) Institutionalized dehumanization from the top down, whereby otherwise ordinary citizens simply did not perceive clients (usually institutional residents) as human, and therefore instituted and upheld systematically abusive practices. This third form of abuse is still extremely common; interestingly, it is this institutionalized abuse by social policy that is the least recognized of the three. Also, it is often at the root of the first type of abuse.

However, the new form of abuse that has been emerging lately, and of which we are bound to see more, is extremely symbolic, and expressive of the dynamics of our times. Not that such abuse has never existed before, but it is now, for the first time, reaching proportions and symbolism commensurate with its newer larger significance. It may be perpetrated not by otherwise cruel people, and not by well-meaning but merely ill-informed or even indifferent people, but by people who are driven by deeply seated unconscious dynamics to act out and express larger cultural beliefs, attitudes and trends in regard to non-health, non-beauty, non-power, and the meaning and value of human life. Indeed, this type of abuse may be acted out as much by fellow clients as by human service workers.

What are the new and symbolic forms of abuse? A few examples will follow.

In 1976, three residents at the Pennhurst Institution for the retarded in Pennsylvania were branded with a red hot key, believed to have been done by an employee. Only a few days later, someone who had the keys to the water controls turned on the water on a resident in a bathtub and drowned him, quite possibly by pushing the person's face under water. Brandings are becoming more common generally, and seem to precede even grosser violence.

Deeply symbolic is the remarkable phenomenon that Dr. Volpe himself, one of the world's experts on certain forms of behavior modification, supervised the administration of severe electric shock of up to 2,000 volts over 14 days in order to keep a boy from vomiting, and from digging at his rectum. A total of 3,550 shocks were administered which inflicted 35 burns on the boy's buttocks. One of the symbolic things here is the fact that the voltage started at the level which is usually successful with most people, but that the neglect and rejection that had been inflicted upon this boy by his society had made him into a creature that could make a fool of our most advanced intellectual technology so that even extreme escalation of voltage failed.

Another resident at Pennhurst has been recorded to have been assaulted 143 times, both by other residents and employees.

The vignettes of assaults upon retarded people in the community, and of rapes of retarded women, are increasing. We even are hearing of cases of abduction and torture, some resulting in death. For instance, in Omaha, a retarded young couple living in an apartment with a counselor were abducted by three reportedly non-handicapped citizens who each raped the young woman, and forced both of them to commit various other sexual acts.

Symbolic and mass forms of abuse, while heavily directed at the retarded, are also on the increase toward other impaired groups who offend the values of a hedonistic culture. These events are not readily perceived to be part of a larger pattern, for several reasons. Firstly, they are reported in the local rather than national news media, Secondly, few people are mentally prepared to believe that patterns of abuse are in the making.

When legalization of euthanasia comes, it will come in the name of six favorite deceptions and disguises. They will say (as I can clearly document) that putting a person to death is good medicine and good science. The second disguise will be mercy, love, humanism and honesty. Thirdly, religion: re-member that Satan pretends to be God. This is his favorite disguise at all times. So we will be, and have been, told that it is good Christianity to put people to death. The fourth one is the denial of the value of life, the claim that certain lives are not worthy, perhaps invoking cost-benefit issues. Fifthly, of course, and maybe the most obvious one, is the denial of humanness of a person and that, therefore, murder will not be murder. Sixthly, euthanasia will be good law. It is essential that we should recognize those six signs, because they have much persuasive power.

IMPLICATIONS OF THE PROPHETIC MESSAGE
OF THE MENTALLY RETARDED

The above events are not isolated. The same thing seems to be happening not just within the l'Arche context from which I have drawn many of my examples, but also within other contexts. Other people are observing the same thing, but to date, such observations have not been well collated and more widely shared and discussed.

That retarded people are carrying prophetic messages has hopeful, glori-ous, but simultaneously frightening messages. What is going on? Why are retarded people achieving world-wide importance at this time, and especially so within the context of a religious movement? In the whole history of humanity, I am not aware of such a pattern of prophetic events having oc-curred before, or having been recorded, shared, and interpreted.

In order to better fathom this phenomenon, I have, during the last few years, looked deeply into the history of mental retardation, and especially into some of the less explored recesses of that history, trying to find out whether there had been earlier public major prophetic appearances of re-tarded people. I was able to identify at most two phenomena that might conceivably qualify. One was that of the historical role of many retarded persons as "jesters" of the high-placed, especially during the Middle Ages;

and secondly, a chain of episodes in the late 1700s and early 1800s, involving "Wild Peter of Hanover," the "Wild Boy of Aveyron," and Caspar Hauser. Interestingly, this chain of events coincided with the rise of the modern Enlightenment–the very thing that we now see the end-result of: the materialism, scientism and technology of today. Thus, at that time of major intellectual transition, there were some appearances of retarded people that might have been of a prophetic nature (elaborated in the appendix to this paper).

In essence, I have already indicated several major implications of these signs and messages. Here, I will restate or elaborate four of them.

The Bankruptcy of Intellectual and Technological Achievement

A passage of fascinating relevance to the little people of the world occurs in Luke 10. Christ had sent out 72 disciples "like lambs among wolves," who returned exulting later because of all the things (healing, etc.) they had found themselves being able to do in his name, including even the casting out of devils even though Christ had not instructed them to exorcise as he had them to teach, preach and cure. In response to the disciples' reports, Christ exclaimed that he "saw Satan fall like lightning from heaven"–and he "rejoiced in the Holy Spirit." This is the only time the Bible made a specific reference to his rejoicing, and the cause of it was probably not only the fall of Satan but the fact that the report of the 72 had made clear that things which were not intellectually accessible to bright and learned people had been revealed to little ones–mere babes. Thus, we must expect no less today, i.e., that some truths will be manifested by or through the little people of this age, even though the same truths escape the world of important people. If God is suddenly elevating retarded people to special and worldwide prominence, we may be witnessing the ultimate instance of God choosing the foolish to confound the wise, and there must be a terribly important message. He must be laughing in divine humor at mankind's intellectual pretensions and achievements. I think that He is telling us that intellect, and the products of intellect (namely, science and technology in the broadest sense) are bankrupt and are about to be foreclosed: when these are cut loose from the Spirit, it is the end of the line for them. Perhaps we are being told that the technology which our intellect has so proudly produced is about to destroy us–as well it can; and/or that He is about to bring the age of modernism to a gruesome end.

Along these lines, I am reminded of the metaphor of the human versus the divine city. In allusion to Genesis 4:14 ("Cain was the founder of a city," i.e., the first city), the poet Robert Lowell wrote:

When Cain
Beat out his brother Abel's brain
The Lord laid down great cities in his soul.

The city, then, was a symbol of sinful mankind striking out on its own, as it was once more later with Babel (Genesis 11: "let us build ourselves a city"), with Sodom and Gomorrah, with Nineveh, and with the timeless and place-less Babylon of the Apocalypse. Ellul (*The Meaning of the City*, 1970) simi-larly takes the city that Cain built as a paradigm of all humanly constructed cities, which have become powers which humans seem incapable of control-ling or directing. Indeed, it is the phenomenon of the uncontrollable technolo-gized and immoralized city that now controls and directs entire societies.

In discerning the divine message of our intellectual bankruptcy, let us also recall that in prophetic manifestations involving the lame, the lepers, the blind and other afflicted persons, they were restored to functioning, and the dead were restored to life. In contrast, the mentally retarded, in their prophet-ic manifestations today, are not being "healed" by being granted brilliance and worldly accomplishment: they are "only" being endowed and bestowed with valued presence, and in some instances–with wisdom.[3] It used to be that when the afflicted person came to Jesus, he said "Take up your bed and walk," and by golly you walked. We do not say to the retarded, "Pick up your marbles and think!" And yet, there is something of very fundamental value and, simultaneously, to me at least, terror-inspiring as well as hopeful in the prophetic phenomena we are witnessing. How bad must things be, how low must the human spirit have sunk, when with our brilliance, learning, and science we can go to the moon, cross the Atlantic in three hours, and do other incredible things, and yet it is those who are deficient in reason and judgment, in rationality, foresight and planning, those who are valued by no society, who are being elevated to such prophetic importance and are being given the mandate for prophecy at the very moment when human intellect has soared to incomprehensibly high achievements. What awful things there must be going on around us! On the other side of the coin, how hopeful is the promise if one can accept the futility of "disembodied" (i.e., cut loose from the Spirit) secular accomplishment. The message must be that all those kinds of works are like the proverbial grass of the Old Testament: up in the morning, gone at night, blown with the wind like the graven images and the false gods. We might say that the titanium of the SST and of the space capsules has replaced the gold of the golden calf, and that the roles of the SST, space capsules and other technological feats are not only that of idols, but that they will disap-pear as such as well–although much like the marvelous mechanical idol of the Moloch, they may devour many people, much as the modern death ma-chines called nursing homes are doing today.

But a word of warning now on what I am saying: I am not saying in all of this that intellect or intellectualism is bad, and that you have to reject it. We are always meant to use our faculties, but of course only in obedience and subservience to the Spirit. But when intellect is cut loose from the Spirit, or even seeks dominance over the Spirit, then it becomes a most powerful force for Evil.

The Importance of Shared Worship with Retarded People

The signs of prophecy have special implications to the people in religious affairs. One implication in all of this is that the retarded people must be related to as partners in the Faith.

After all, if the Lord has chosen the retarded to be his prophets, then they must be viewed as partners, not as a group of pagans to be converted and colonized, or even as a group of children to be catechized. There must be less glorification of the now almost technological-mechanistic religious education of the handicapped by people who see themselves as in possession of the spiritual goods. In the mainstream church, this is one of the major problems, because the major focused vehicle of relationship to the retarded in the churches tends to be colonization. "We" are bright and learned, "we" have got all the catechism and knowledge, "we" have the Bible and its interpretation, and "we" are going to have to come and colonize the retarded people who are stupid and religiously ignorant. "We" must "reach the retarded": let's go, grab them! Not "they reach us," but "we reach them." That is the message I get over, and over, and over, and over, including in the preoccupation with religious education by many members of the Religion Division of the American Association on Mental Deficiency, and by many other pastoral personnel.

Religious education is important, and I am not advising against it. But it must not be the major medium. Much of this type of "religious colonization" reminds me of the olden days where they converted the heathens, and the first thing they did was to make sure they wore clothing, then they made them work for wages, and then they taught them all the vices of our society–and 30 years later, the natives had a cultural and societal collapse because they had learned all of our vices. That is why I call it colonization–colonizing the retarded with religious empires.

We must make a fundamental reappraisal of the relative importance we have assigned not only to all formal religious education, but also of the relative importance of retarded people as compared to non-retarded people in religious life generally. There is vastly more to religious life than religious education. Religious education is only a means, a technology towards a goal, not the goal itself. Instead, there has got to be more emphasis on shared worship, and shared prayer. This issue calls for a heightened commitment to, and ingenuity in, finding ways of enlarging the meaningful worship participation of retarded people.

Just before I gave a version of this address for the first time (to the Religion Division of the American Association on Mental Deficiency), somebody asked me, "What are you going to talk about?" Being on the run, I shouted, "in a nutshell, get off the religious education kick and get on the worship kick." That is only one way of putting it, if one is a bit crude about it. Even in shared worship, we have to orient ourselves to genuine religious sharing, and not the condescending sharing that I see so much of. In genuine sharing, the retarded person is not just said to be equal at the communion rail and so on, but the equality is experienced, is real. The worship structure is such as to communicate it, and the events are such as to manifest it. When the social environment of worship is properly prepared, then prophecy will find its place; we will experience it. We are apt not to witness it when we come in and colonize, as the superior ambassadors from the other planet of intellect and reading that is so important, as implied in many of our religious education approaches, curricula, publications, etc. The sharing has got to be genuine, not contrived. There must be genuine contributive roles for retarded people in integrated worship and religious life, and not just in our own segregated human service settings, not just in our institutions and religious education contexts, but in our group homes, and certainly and foremost in the congregational life of our churches. Retarded people must have genuine roles in ordinary, normative mainstream religious life. It may take some thinking as to how to make it genuine, so it is not contrived, phony, catastrophic or ridiculing. Even if someone did laugh, it does not mean that it is inherently of a derisive nature; also, the person who laughs today may learn something tomorrow.

Also, the sharing must be expressed in the language. The "we" versus "they" language which permeates the religious education literature has got to go. It is always the "us" and the "them" which comes up over and over, and which would not be found in a genuine sharing approach to religious worship; "we" reaching or doing something for "them" when, in fact, if the prophecy that I have posited above is true, it is the other way around. The Lord is trying to "reach us" through "them," trying to give us a message: "Without my presence, the brain doesn't work! It's no good! Technology is bringing the end. Cataclysm, destruction–that is where all the brains are leading. Just listen." But we are too busy beating catechism or even Bible stories into retarded people to listen.[4] We are too retarded, too blind, and too deaf to get the message.

In fact, one may ask further whether there is not an unconscious immorality in many (not necessarily all) forms of religious education and religious participation that are segregated. There might be hypocrisy in such segregated activities in that religious education is used as yet another endorsement of societal rejection of its unwanted or low-value members. My guess is that willfully imposed segregated religious activities are theologically unsound unless all other options and methods have been exhausted first. Indeed, the segregation that is often imposed or glorified by the world should not merely be rejected by Christian allies of the retarded, but should be confronted both by the word and in prophetic action, and what better way to accomplish this than in the Christian churches, worship, and instruction. Oddly enough, I find it almost impossible to conceive of a situation where integration would fail if it were conducted in commitment to the Spirit. Such a failure would probably tell us that the particular congregation or setting is no longer a religious one, but one masquerading as such–though quite likely unconsciously.

One of Stringfellow's (1973) major messages is that human institutions, and indeed all of natural creation, are fallen. We tend to think of human beings as fallen creatures, but this book says no, not just human beings, but human institutions too are fallen; they have an identity of their own that transcends that of their individual members. Since they are fallen, they are by nature non-functional: they naturally tend toward corruption, decay and evil. Indeed, Stringfellow says, human institutions are "principalities and powers," and they tend toward idolatry, because fallen humans tend to elevate secular forms into what amounts to divine stature and worship.

After I read Stringfellow's compelling reasoning and documentation, I began to see the world in a whole new pattern. I became much more pessimistic about the effectiveness of worldly planning, organizing and service structuring. I began to see idolatry where I had never seen it before. For instance, after reading this book, I began to see idolatry in churches. I can never again go into a church, see a national flag sitting next to the altar, and not shudder. Suddenly, I perceive the idolatry, because the placement of the flag equates the secular nation with the City of God, the heavenly chosen, the Jerusalem of on high. The secular nation is the fallen Babylon (e.g., Revelation 18-19), and it is always the Babylon, at all times, and in all places. It is a Babylon which at times is a little worse than others, and sometimes more clear-cut than at others. But it still is Babylon, and it is of this earth, and it captures and controls more people than does the City of God, and it makes them do bad things! It makes them ill, and it legitimizes it; it makes them reject other people; and so on.

States and nations, cities, the secular law, the police, universities, voluntary associations, clubs, professional or parent groups in mental retardation, corporations, firms, businesses, and to some degree, and in a certain sense, even the churches–they all are principalities and powers. In a sense, at the moment and to the degree that the church becomes humanly organized, it becomes a power and a principality, a human organization with human rules, penalties, and so on. In a sense, human institutions are not only inclined to evil the same as individual persons, Stringfellow points out, but even more so, because the principalities and the powers are more evil and more inclined to evil than even people. After all, there are such things as saintly people, but there are no such things as saintly organizations, countries, armies, political parties, business firms, or professional organizations.

This is how the institution of the church can become the fallen human institution: the moment when it is formalized organizationally. I think the evidence from history surely bears up this point. A fascinating observation of Stringfellow's is that whereas the moral authority of God can be expressed in many ways–through grace, revelations, miracles, healing, prophecy, absolute power, limits, fiats, and ultimately in damnation or salvation–the ultimate secular authority, e.g., that of the state, is only one: it is merely death. That is the only ultimate moral authority of the state. Death can be partial, via imprisonment and torture: or it can be the real death of the body.

Stringfellow's insight permits us to understand why persons who have freed themselves from the fear of death can defy the power of an evil earthly authority in serenity and freedom. Not surprisingly, it is these very persons who arouse the ire of earthly authority the most, because they have escaped it. That explains so many remarkable phenomena of people being persecuted out of all proportion to their offenses. We do not understand it until, I think, we understand this. Then we say, ah-ha, often these are the people who have escaped the moral authority of the state, having escaped the moral authority of death. Evil then becomes fanatic, frantic and aroused. So we read about someone like Daniel in the lion's pit, the Maccabees, the early Christians in the arena who had all risen above death; we see the Berrigans who have aroused ire far beyond the ridiculous little symbolic things they have done, such as burning draft cards, digging graves in the White House lawn, or deftly chaining shut the Pentagon doors. The only thing that makes these ridiculous gestures so incredibly offensive is that they reveal that their enactors have escaped from (risen above?) the moral authority of the state. People like that bring forth the ire of the children of darkness out of all proportion to the secular offensiveness of the acts.

Ever since I encountered and believed Stringfellow's analysis, I have abandoned my faith in the power of secular moral service structures. This does not mean that I do not believe that we must try to moralize secular service structures, but that we must count our successes as either being illusory as, for example, when winning litigative victories in courts; or as minor, where we can casually accept some developments as little victories, but not as being a big deal; or at best, as being temporary and transient in the scope of things even when it is a real and big victory. In a few years, the natural dynamics of the principalities and powers will again triumph in the secular realm, and again the system will regress to low functionality–at least by any Jerusalem-type of standard.

At any rate, these reflections are meant to underline that Satanic deception, perversion, and even idolatry must be expected to be found even within churches, and that "good intentions" are not enough of a base for constructive relations between church and retarded people. If the good intentions are not accompanied by something else that is very much of the Spirit, then they may indeed pave the road to hell, as the English proverb has it.

The Importance of Other Genuine Sharing with Retarded People

Stringfellow's analysis made it clear to me that the Holy Spirit detests organization. This does not mean that we can live without organization; especially as human congregations increase, humans will increasingly organize. However, it does mean that the Spirit is more apt to move where people try to live by the guidance of the Spirit rather than by formalistic means, by organized planning, etc.

In the Faust drama by Goethe, Faust hears Easter church bells ringing and soliloquizes (roughly translated): "Oh, yes, the message I do hear–but I lack faith." I believe that most Christians suffer from that condition to various extents. We hear the message that calls for surrender to the Spirit, for accepting insecurity and what to us appears as disorder, but we can hardly believe our senses that such a thing should be called for, and for this reason and others, we cling to the security of all kinds of formalizations and organization. Ironically, and predictably, organized functioning turns out to eventuate in chaos–as it has to, being what it is, i.e., fallen, and under the domination of the "Prince of this World." But no matter; we still adhere to various forms of formalistic security.

Considering therefore the fallenness of nature and of formal human organizations, I now see much more importance in informal human ties and relationships. As Stringfellow points out, the church is like a flame which flickers up more intensely and informally in some place, and then moves and flickers more intensively elsewhere as formalism takes over. The real Pentecostal church is not found in huge, formal organization, but in transitory groups and unexpected phenomena; it is fragile, because it resists organization–yet humans organize by reflex. Therefore, the church of Christ comes, goes, moves; and, of course, finds its expression in different ways in different societies and in different places.

So now, I attach vastly more importance to informal human helping forms and relationships between mentally retarded and non-retarded people, as in non-formalized communal living. Even group homes are almost all formal, incorporated structures, with staff, this and that formal funding, evaluations, reports–fine, but theologically, more important than such formal structures are the informal ones: people living together in a house, unincorporated, unfunded, life-sharing, Pentecostal. Remember Acts 5: they shared things in common, and anyone who had any want received from those who possessed more. That I see as of terribly deep importance at this time. I would not go so far as to say that members of informal communities today should not accept generic pensions, such as Social Security; but I would prefer it if community living came about not through formal organizations, but through the informal, prophetic and Pentecostal way. Of course, I do not expect that to be a major secular service system solution; I do not expect this to be a quantitative solution for the need of vast numbers of retarded people, but I see it as a qualitative, way-pointing prophetic manifestation.

Perhaps we need to distinguish between what we believe and what we know we will end up doing that violates our belief; and between the weaknesses of two imperfect, fallen helping forms: the formal organized helping form will almost certainly deteriorate to perversion and/or abuse; the informal human helping is more apt to terminate and be unstable. What drives us to insist that stability is worth more than the benefits of informality, and more worth the risk of deterioration to abuse than the risk of discontinuity? I submit that the issue deserves deep, drawn-out thought rather than easy dismissal.

Those Allied with Severely Handicapped People Must Be Prepared to Be Persecuted and Martyred

Of course, if severely handicapped people will be persecuted, those who stand with them will be subject to the same onslaught. In turn, this means that those who align themselves with this potential target of destruction must be willing to accept martyrdom as well. Many times, standing nearly alone with a cause that will have no or little rational secular defense may be much greater suffering than death itself. In fact, it is conceivable that the martyrdom of the non-handicapped defenders of the handicapped will often not consist of death but of scorn; vilification; social exile; denial of education, employment, and professional status; impoverishment; etc. Many defenders will only be able to stand up if they are part of small mutual support communities.

To conclude: among my recent historical studies, I have been exploring the history of how several hundreds of thousands of handicapped and retarded people were exterminated in Nazi Germany. At the German institutions, gray buses would pull up and people would be called up and stamped with a number on their hand, just as in the Apocalypse, the Beast stamped its mark on its victims. The mark was the sign of death. The victims would be put into a bus with painted-over windows so that no one could look in or out, and driven off, supposedly to "relocation centers" which actually were extermination centers. For a long time, people could not be sure of what was happening, because it was all done so deceptively. You were only told that there was relocation, congregation of people with different conditions, and so on. But in time, enough evidence emerged so that moral people could come to the judgment that handicapped people were being destroyed. At that point, several (mostly Protestant) pastors decided to stand in the door, and said to the Hitlers, "Before you take another one of my people, you must take me." It was a risk that had little likelihood of succeeding, yet at that time in the war, the German leadership felt that it was politically too touchy to open yet another "front" by putting too many respected pastors in the concentration camp, and so the remnants of retarded people were saved.

I have already said that those who stand with the mentally retarded people must be prepared to be martyred. It may not come to that, but one must be prepared for it nevertheless. So the question is: should our era's version of that day come, will I, first of all, have the discernment to know where they are taking the mentally retarded? Each age has its own metaphorical expression. What are the executioners going to look like in this age when they come? Maybe they are dressed in white instead of black, and instead of military ranks, they may have medical ones. Maybe they will take the mentally retarded to nursing homes instead of concentration camps or sanitoria. Whatever will be the metaphor for extermination of our age, it will call for discernment. And then I may have to figure out what is happening to the retarded, where they are being martyred, and how; and once I can discern that, the next question is whether I will have the courage to stand in the door.

After an unsuccessful previous attempt, an unknown assailant succeeded in 1833 in stabbing to death, under mysterious circumstances, Caspar Hauser on a street in Ansbach, Germany (see Appendix to this article). The reason this event is of great importance is that there exists sufficient credible documentation to believe that Hauser had been made mentally retarded by environmental deprivation during childhood, and then been made unretarded by environmental stimulation during adolescence. On Hauser's tombstone, he was called an *"aenigma sui temporis,"* i.e., an enigma of his time.

Do not the phenomena recited in this chapter pose an enigma for our time? The enigma of the retarded person in an age of intellect and high technological development and excellence is heightened by the curious phenomenon that it is precisely at this time in history at which seriously impaired persons are increasingly being defined out of the human race, that animals are beginning to be defined as sharing with human beings intelligence and related characteristics that previously were viewed as being uniquely human. Thus, we now read of experiments with chimpanzees that prove that they have sufficient linguistic skills to write meaningful communicative sentences, using symbol systems somewhat along the lines of ideographs. We witness phenomena such as expensive pet grooming shops, commercial whorehouses for pets, and expensive pet cemeteries with all the human trimmings. The money spent on pet foods, pet clothing, and other pet paraphernalia runs into hundreds of millions of dollars annually, giving human services for the mentally retarded a respectable "run for its money." *Aenigma nostri temporis* (an enigma of *our* time).

A CONCLUDING PERSONAL NOTE

Several friends who read the earlier drafts of this paper suggested that I define more clearly what I mean by "prophecy." It so happens that I am a person who is obsessed with organization, planning, precision, etc.–exactly all the things the Spirit usually flees from, as pointed out above. However, for once, my being strongly rebels against precision. I am deeply wondered by the fact that God has graced me with the gift of perceiving the prophetic manifestation and role of mentally retarded people, and I want to preserve my sense of puzzled wide-eyedness, wonderment, and openness to the unexpected, intangible, and poorly definable. I am almost afraid that if I become too precise, the "thing" might slip away from me. So I must ask the reader for forgiveness for indulging in a bit of vagueness. I always thought that if medieval theologians had not been so definition-crazy, the church would have been a happier one.

*   *   *

At the conference where this presentation was first given, the speaker invited the participants to contribute as follows:

I ask you now to share prophetic signs, to think of instances where you may have witnessed prophecy that took place either by handicapped people, or mediated through handicapped people, that have manifested the glory of God either in public acts, or in dispelling evil, or in gentling, or in healing, or in tongues, or in the dance of the Lord, or in any other manifestations that you may have witnessed.

One of the participants, a nun who teaches retarded children:

> This is a very small incident that occurred on Ash Wednesday. It involved a 15-year old child in my class whom I was trying to prepare for first Holy Communion the past 5 or 6 years, and finally he consented. Before communion, I had prayed spontaneously with him and he followed right along. After communion, when he returned back to his place, he started to pray spontaneously by himself. This may seem like a small thing, but ordinarily his speech was one or two words, but here, he used complete sentences. It was just beautiful. I could not pray with him because it was so . . . it just filled up, it touched me so. I never thought too much about it, until this morning. I really feel that the Lord had given him the gift of tongues after he had received communion. And another thing: I could never get him to say the word of Jesus. If I asked him who

he would like to receive, he always said "God." His mother was not present, by the way, because this was a very spontaneous thing the way it happened. After he had received, she asked, "Who did you receive this morning, Bill?" and he said, "Jesus." That in itself, I thought was so touching, so I am very happy to praise the Lord for the whole thing.

Another participant:

I have been very concerned with bringing the Eucharist to the profoundly disabled. In the past couple of months, I met a 50-year old man with Down's syndrome who had never received the Eucharist. He had very little speech. His sister was really the only one who could understand him. He kept telling me what his name was, and it was John. He was very happy when I suggested to his sister that he receive the Eucharist. I went once to his house and I took all of the things with me that the priest uses. I had no idea whether he knew what I was saying, but I just presented these things to him, like "This is the kind of bread the priest uses," and so on. He would smile in a distracted way, but I had no idea whether he was comprehending any of the things I was saying. And then I said, "John, would you like to go to church?" I took him to his parish because I wanted him to be comfortable with the physical surroundings. We went up to the tabernacle in the church, and I said to John, "This is where Jesus is in this special way. Would you like to touch the tabernacle?" And John, who had been all smiles, he looked at me seriously, and his hands started to tremble. He laid his trembling hands in front of the tabernacle and he started to cry . . . just tears, such a cry . . . and I thought, how could anyone say more eloquently, "This is Jesus."

Another participant:

We have a girl in our program named Rosy. She is in a wheelchair, and she always tells us exactly what is on her mind, and what she thinks. For instance, at a gathering, if no one is talking to Rosy, she says, "Are you here? Do you know that I am here?" When her priest heard that she was in our program, he said, "You know, that is a great idea. Maybe we can start this in our parish. I've got to get to know Rosy, so that we can start this." So he began coming to visit Rosy every week. For the first three weeks, Rosy would not speak to him. The third week, he said, "Rosy, I know you can talk. Why won't you talk to me?" And she said, "My brother and sister went to your church. But you had nothing for me. They went to your Sunday school. You did not have a place for me. You taught them about God, and I wanted to know. You had nothing for me. Now, I went and found my own church. Now, you come and say that you want to start something for me. Go home, damn priest." She was telling him, and all of us, exactly where we are at.

Another participant:

Retarded children really can and do express an understanding of the sacraments. One was a little child who was baptized, and the priest had her turn to the congregation and everybody was clapping–and she gave the sign of victory.

Another young fellow received the Eucharist for the first time. What he did was symbolic of what the Eucharist is. The priest gave him the host and then he shouted, "Thank you, Father," and then he grabbed the priest around the waist and gave him the biggest hug. The priest could do nothing but put the chalice down and hug him back.

APPENDIX

THE APPARENTLY FIRST WORLD-WIDE PUBLICITY OF RETARDED PERSONS

Above, I indicated that with one previous exception, I was not aware of any other patterns of world-wide visibility of retarded persons. To clarify this point, and also in order to provide potential support to some of the above speculations concerning the theological meaning of retarded persons, I briefly reviewed the relevant historical facts, leaning especially on Singh and Zingg (1939), and Lane (1976).

Some retarded people may have occupied relatively public roles as "professional fools" (court fools, jester, etc.) from earliest times. However, any such individual was apt to become known to only a limited circle of people, and/or only locally. The apparently first record of a retarded jester acquiring international "prominence" involved Claus Narr, the court fool who "belonged" to Duke Frederick the Wise of Saxony (1463-1525). (Narr means fool, and thus his role became his last name.) Of similar "fame" was Triboulet (early to mid-1500s), the jester of King Francis I of France (1494-1547), whose portraits reveal him to have had classical microcephaly. While Triboulet's fame was modest, his image became world famous because Victor Hugo made a major (though distorted) role for him in his novel *Le Roi S'Amuse* (sometimes translated as *The King's Dalliance*); and in a yet further distortion of his true identity, he became immortal as a major figure in Verdi's opera *Rigoletto*.

Not long later, Jeppe, a retarded dwarf with minimal speech became known to many people in Europe because he was the household fool of the most famous astronomer of his age, Tycho Brahe (1546-1601), who traveled widely and worked for the courts of several European countries. The dwarf attracted special attention because Brahe thought that he was able (presumably because of divine favor) to reveal hidden truths and the future (Dryer, 1963; Gade, 1947).

Aside from these limited forerunners, really major public visibility of retarded people occurred as a result of religious, philosophic, and scientific interest in the innate nature of human beings. The question that had preyed on the minds of thinkers for millennia was what human beings were naturally really like, and the only way to find out was to examine humans who had not been contaminated by the process of human socialization. This meant that any children or adults who could be found who had been raised without human contact would be very valuable for study.

Accounts of children raised by animals go back to the early mythology of many cultures; one only needs to recall the story of Romulus and Remus, and that in American Indian legends, the first humans were wolves. However, the concept and even term of "feral man" was apparently coined by Carl Linnaeus (1707-1778) (although Triboulet's original name was said to have been Le Ferial, according to Senelick and Yenne, 1977) who defined a *homo sapiens ferus* in his early great work *Systema Naturae* (1735).

There had been isolated early accounts of children reared by animals, and these stories probably attracted as much but no more attention than any number of other curiosities of a world hungry for diversion from the humdrum of everyday life. Many such stories might have been fueled by the custom, even quite early, of exhibiting people of unusual appearance or behavior for money, and inducing (or even forcing) them into unnatural behavior in order to make them more newsworthy. Also, physically deformed, mentally deranged and mentally retarded people have been characteristically highly at risk of being likened to animals, being animal-imaged, and being literally treated as animals, or worse. Linnaeus specifically cited nine famous cases reported and recorded between 1344 and 1731, including the "Hessian Wolf Boy" and "Wild Peter of Hanover." The thread was eagerly taken up by Jean Jacques Rousseau whose *Origins of Inequality* appeared in 1755, because it was consistent with his concept of the noble savage.

Practically all the descriptions of feral children or "wild" people are applicable to mentally retarded or severely emotionally disturbed (e.g., "autistic") individuals. It is quite likely that many of them had been abandoned or gotten lost, and might have been at liberty only a few days or even hours before being "found." Of course, if someone had abandoned them, they were not too likely to step forward and reclaim them, particularly since a handicapped child was much better off in the public limelight and under the care of well-to-do people who usually became their patrons than in the homes of humble folk.

A whole series of "wild boy" discoveries specifically seemed to have had its origin with Wild Peter of Hanover who was discovered in the fields of the German town of Hamel in 1724, although inadequate attention is usually given to the fact that a fragment of a shirt was still fastened around his neck. The case came to the attention of King George I (of Hanover and Britain) because of the prevailing interest in the theory of natural development, and with a great deal of publicity in various court and intellectual circles, Peter was eventually transported to Britain. He was deemed important enough that at least two portraits of him have come down to us. He was eventually placed under the care of a farmer in Hertfordshire where he died in old age in 1758.

The next major figure in this genealogy of "wild" figures was the "Wild Boy of Aveyron." The accounts of the initial contacts with the Wild Boy, as in many of these stories of "wild" children, are remarkably inconsistent. According to some sources that sound very credible to me, he was seen in the woods of Southern France as early as 1795, was "found" in about 1797, was seen in the woods later in 1797 and was caught again in 1798, escaped once more, was caught in 1799, escaped, and then voluntarily entered a house hungry and cold in January of 1800.

Cross-checking in Lane's (1976) new classic on the boy, he was still able to speak a little in 1798, and I find it remarkable that one of the few things he could say was that his father was "Donne á Dieu" (give to God; maybe he meant 'donné á Dieu, i.e., given to God'); and during his 1798 captivity, he had been publicly put on display in the city square of Lacaune. Prior to his 1800 house entry, he had actually entered and been fed in many houses, and had been seen swimming or bathing in the streams. Also, he had four facial scars, and one apparently severe throat scar.

Just how well-informed even modestly educated people of the enlightenment period were is not widely appreciated today. Upon the Wild Boy's discovery, numerous people (perhaps more than would be the case today) immediately recognized the scientific importance of the event, and strove to utilize the opportunity for experimentation which, informal and spontaneous as it was, was often quite ingenious, as was also true later with Caspar Hauser.

Very quickly, by summer 1800, the boy had been brought to a young physician-educator, Itard, in Paris (catching smallpox on the way), who named him "Victor," which means "he who is victorious." By 1803, Victor had achieved quite a bit of publicity, and even more so by 1828 (when he died, aged approximately 40) because of the interest of the intellectual world of that age in the nature-nurture controversy, and its implications to politics and government. In the early 1970s, a film was made about him ("Wild Child," directed by François Truffaut).

Lane also points out a special irony in Victor entering world publicity as "The wild[5] boy[6] of Aveyron," so that few people even recall his name as "Victor." Victor was not savage, he was not a child-infant but an adolescent, and he was not even from the Department of Aveyron (there is apparently no town by that name), but from the Department of Tarn.

In the same year Victor died, Caspar Hauser appeared mysteriously in 1828 on the streets of Nuremberg at the estimated age of 17, with the reported mentality of a 3 year old, and with a letter in his hand addressed to the commander of a local cavalry unit. He was able to speak only a few stereotyped words–but significantly, he spoke them in what appeared to be Bavarian dialect. Also, he was reported to have been able to write his name rather readily even the very day he was discovered. *He apparently became one of the most famous persons who were retarded*–even though some people would deny his retardation because he overcame his stunted mental development in many ways. Incredibly, thousands of pamphlets, documentary books, novels, and even plays were–and still are–written about him (including a recent film, "Every Man for Himself and God Against All"). He remained a controversial figure or symbol in public affairs until the end of the German principalities in 1918, when World War I ended. He was said to have been the most famous person in Europe, aside perhaps from some of the major European rulers. He was not only proclaimed by Nüremberg as a "child of the city," but became known by the remarkable title of "the child of Europe." One of the major theories was that he was the heir of the House of Baden, a principality in the southwest corner of Germany. Soon after he gained publicity, an attempt to assassinate him was made, apparently after it was advertised that he was writing his memoirs–which later proved to be nothing more than a few pages of vague recollections of his earlier life in a dungeon-like setting. After only five years of public life, he was stabbed to death by an unknown assassin in 1833 in Ansbach (northern Bavaria), and is buried under a gravestone with a famous inscription.[7]

Hauser was described as mild, obedient, and good natured, with great aversion to meat, coffee, or any kind of alcoholic beverage. He appeared to have no form of religious conceptualization at all despite the bizarre fact that his pockets were full of religious tracts when he was discovered. Apparently, when he first saw a life-size crucifix on the outside of a church, he was seized with horror and pain, and pleaded that the man that was so dreadfully tormented might be taken down. Another most fascinating aspect of this case is the fact that Hauser referred to the shadowy male adult who had been his keeper during his dimly recollected childhood as "the man with whom I always was."

Interestingly, Hauser apparently had focal seizures for some time, associated with his initial sensitivity to light. He may also have had petit mal and/or autonomic seizures, and/or possible allergies to all kinds of animal and plant substances. The latter hypothesis would not be too far-fetched if he had spent years of his childhood in a sheltered and possibly dust-free setting (i.e., a dungeon or cellar). Hauser also displayed many of the characteristics of autistic children. He had a passion for order; referred to himself and other people by their name instead of with pronouns; had initially an almost photographic memory; had a preoccupation with what he considered to be dirt or dust; and attributed intelligence and will to inanimate objects, and human sentiment to animals.

I strongly suspect that Hauser was exactly what the letter in his hand said: the illegitimate child of a servant girl and a cavalry man somewhere along the border of Bavaria and Austria, perhaps in the Regensburg or Munchen (Munich) area. I also suspect that he had had some normal child-rearing, and then had been confined later in a dark basement or attic room where he lost some of his earlier growth, but regained it with the stimulation received during his years of liberty. For instance, with only minimal training, he is said to have ridden a horse better than many people with extensive prior training. I would also not be surprised if he had not actually been younger than his suspected 17 years, and therefore perhaps more responsive to education.

The speculations about his origins probably arose from the romantic imagination of a sensation-hungry age. Indeed, the ascription of a secret noble birth to foundlings, etc., was very common in that day (e.g., Lane, 1976, p. 322), as we can perhaps also infer from the fairy tales of those days that have come down to us, including even the themes of the prince-as-frog. Even the theater of that day was full of plays of unidentified noble children.

Of considerable interest is exactly who first spawned the hypothesis of Hauser's noble descent. If it was his first mentor, the prominent politician, Anselm Ritter von Feuerbach, as seems likely, one should wonder whether such a hypothesis sprang from a political (though quite likely unconscious) motivation. Feuerbach was a loyal servant of the kingdom of Bavaria, and it is fascinating to trace what Bavaria had to gain if it could be proved that the ruling house of Baden was illegitimate, or involved in a crime. Indeed, daughters of the House of Baden had married into the ruling families of Russia, Austria and Bavaria, all of whom thus had grounds for a claim to the throne of Baden if the legitimate line should die out, as it eventually did. The plot thickens when one considers that the northern part of Baden had at one time been under the rulers of Bavaria. But almost totally ignored seems to have been the possibility that the corrupt rulers of Baden might indeed have instigated Hauser's assassination–not because he was the true heir, but because of the rumors that he was. Thus, in the Machiavellian scheme of things, the assassination would make excellent sense as being "for good measure."

However, none of this is to deny the special symbolism and even message which Caspar constituted, or the fact that "a crime upon the soul-life of a person" had indeed been committed, as said the title of the book about him by his early mentor, Feuerbach.

As in the case of Victor, there is also potential symbolism involving Caspar's name. Caspar (in German, Kaspar) is, among other things, the clever but also socially suspect hero of puppet shows, as well as Gaspar (or Gaspard), the "treasure bringer," one of the three magi.

Thus, only a few years apart, and at a critical historical time hinge, two retarded people made world history. That which made them famous was what is now bringing ruin to the world: the "enlightenment," the beginning of the rejection of the Christian Western tradition in favor of a naturalism, faith in reason, intelligence, and the perfectibility of human beings. All this was occurring as democratic republicanistic thought was toppling the institution of nobility. It seems as if the modern age of the beginning of the end of intellect was ushered in by two prophetic figures–one of them, the more spiritual one, assassinated. He had come from "him with whom I always was," the other, the "victorious one," had come from "Give to God."

ENDNOTES

1. The prophetic power of public profession by retarded people was also described by Shearer (1974) as follows: ". . . people who in the ordinary way of things have few of the normal abilities of self-expression can talk of their faith and pray with a directness and understanding which has an almost prophetic quality."

2. Apparently, David threw off or lost all his clothing while dancing, but despite the presence of women, this was clearly a non-sexualized dance except apparently in the jealous eyes of Michol.

3. Big deal! Even Psalms 19, 8 pointed it out already: "the decree of the Lord is trustworthy, giving wisdom to the simple."

4. Some of the discussion that followed my first presentation of this revealed that there was some misunderstanding of what I meant. I did *not* mean that all catechism is bad, or that "modern" and "Vatican II approaches" were intrinsically good, nor that child-like worship and simple vocabulary is the answer. To sharpen the issue to its almost ludicrous extreme: I am saying that shared worship in Latin, Greek or Sanskrit is more valid if it is "for real," than the most "enlightened" and pedagogic approach that is ultimately derived from, or reflective of, theologically invalid assumptions and stances, or that tries to replace the fervor of worship with the clever elegance of pedagogic technology.

5. "Le sauvage" in French.

6. "L'Enfant" in French.

7. Hiciacet

Casparus Hauser
Aenigma sui temporis
Ignota nativitas
Occulta mors
MD CCC XXXIII

(Here lies Caspar Hauser, an enigma of his time, of unknown birth, and mysterious death 1833.).

REFERENCES

Binding, K., and Hoche, A. (1920). *Die Freigabe der vernichtung Lebensunwerten Lebens: Ihr Mass und Ihre Form.* Leipzig, Germany: Felix Meiner.

Binding, K. and Hoche, A. (1975). *The release of the destruction of life devoid of value.* Santa Ana, CA: Life Quality Paperbacks. (Originally published in 1920 by Felix Meiner, Leipzig, Germany; annotated by Robert L. Sassone).

Deacon, J.J. (1974). *Tongue tied: Fifty years of friendship in a subnormality hospital.* London: National Society for Mentally Handicapped Children.

DeVries-Kruyt, T. *Small ship, great sea: The life story of a mongoloid boy.* London: Collins, 1971. (Published in the U.S. as *A special gift: The story of Jan.* New York: Peter Wyden, 1971).

Dreyer, J.L.E. (1963). *Tycho Brache: A picture of scientific life and work in the sixteenth century.* New York: Dover. (Reproduction: Originally published, 1890, by Adam and Charles Black).

Ellul, J. (1970). *The meaning of the city.* Grand Rapids, MI: Eerdmans.

Gade, J. (1974). *Life and times of Tycho Brahe.* Westport, CT.: Greenwood.

Hong, E. (1976). *Bright valley of love.* Minneapolis: Augsburg Publishing House.

Hunt, N. (1967). *The world of Nigel Hunt: The diary of a mongoloid youth.* New York: Garrent Publications.

Kerr, M.L. *Retarded and happy.* Pratt, KS: The Printing Press (undated).

Lane, H. (1976). *The wild boy of Aveyron.* Cambridge, MA: Harvard University Press.

Morishima, A. (1977). Weaknesses, strengths, or a dual approach? A case for capitalizing on talent. *Education and Training of the Mentally Retarded.* 12(1), 36-41.

Senelick, L., and Yenne, B. (1977). *A cavalcade of clowns.* San Francisco, CA: Bellerophon.

Singh, J.A.L., and Zingg, R.M. (1939). *Wolf children and feral man.* IV. Contributions of the University of Denver. New York: Harper and Bros.

Stringfellow, W. (1973). *An ethic for Christians and other aliens in a strange land.* Waco, TX: Word Books.

An Attempt
Toward a Theology of Social Integration
of Devalued/Handicapped People

Wolf Wolfensberger, PhD

OUTLINE AND INTRODUCTION

Some Baseline Facts About Social Devaluation and Segregation
Pre-Christian Historical Patterns of Segregation/Integration
Historical Patterns of Segregation/Integration in the Christian Tradition
Judeo-Christian Rationales for Integration

> Divine Laws and Commandments
> General Principles of Christian Moral Theology
> The Precedents Set by Christ
> Inference of What Christ Would Likely Have Done Had He Come in
>   This Time and World
> The Examples Set By the Lives of the Great Saints
> Divine Guidance and Revelation in the Here and Now

Implications for the Behavior of Integrators
Are There Any Rationales for Segregation?
Concluding Reflection

This paper was first presented at a symposium on "The Theology of Integration of Handicapped and Other Groups of Devalued People" of the Religion Division of the American Association on Mental Deficiency, June, 1978, Denver.

[Haworth co-indexing entry note]: "An Attempt Toward a Theology of Social Integration of Devalued/ Handicapped People." Wolfensberger, Wolf. Co-published simultaneously in *Journal of Religion, Disability & Health* (The Haworth Pastoral Press, an imprint of The Haworth Press, Inc.) Vol. 4, No. 2/3, 2001, pp. 49-70; and: *The Theological Voice of Wolf Wolfensberger* (ed: William C. Gaventa, and David L. Coulter) The Haworth Pastoral Press, an imprint of The Haworth Press, Inc., 2001, pp. 49-70. Single or multiple copies of this article are available for a fee from The Haworth Document Delivery Service [1-800-342-9678, 9:00 a.m. - 5:00 p.m. (EST). E-mail address: getinfo@haworthpressinc.com].

Unless indicated otherwise, I will use the term "segregation" as referring to the physical distantiation that is *imposed* by one group of people upon another. This includes those forms of segregation that are *clearly* imposed, as well as those forms that are imposed by *hidden* dynamics, and even those patterns in which a person or group claims to choose segregation voluntarily, but where such a choice is only an anticipation of expectable enforced segregation. An example of the latter would be the apparently self-selected segregation of people in racial ghettoes, of elderly people in segregated high-rises, etc.

SOME BASELINE FACTS ABOUT SOCIAL DEVALUATION AND SEGREGATION

In order to deal consciously with the polarity of integration versus segregation, it is necessary to be aware of certain facts and fairly well-established socio-psychological principles. One of these is that there are three major categories of people's response to devalued people: (a) attempts at reversal of the characteristics that make that person devalued in the eyes of the observers (perhaps by habilitation, restoration, etc.) or by redefinition of the devalued characteristics as being no longer deviant; (b) denial or repression of someone's (or some group's) devalued status because the reality is too anxiety-provoking to admit; or (c) transaction of "distantiation," which can take the form of either physical or social distantiation.

Distantiation can be achieved in three major ways:

1. One can put distance between oneself and people that one is not comfortable with, or does not like, by destroying them. This destruction can take the form of actual killing, and history is full of relevant examples. This is the ultimate distantiation, the "final solution."
2. One can create physical distance either by removing the devalued group of people, or by removing oneself. Characteristically, which of the two takes place depends on who has the power. It is usually the powerful people who remove the powerless ones whom they do not like. However, occasionally, a minority removes itself from another group that it dislikes, because the minority does not have enough power to remove the people it dislikes. Some of the self-segregation of the rich falls into this category.
3. One can also create social distance, which is often done when one is incapable of creating physical distance, or when sanctions and morals prohibit physical distance. In such cases, social distance is often created in subtle ways. Devalued individuals may be animalized, their social status may be reduced; or, if nothing else can be done, they are simply not interacted with; and when they are unavoidably present, they are treated as nonentities, nonpersons, and objects.

Let us review some baseline facts about segregation. You cannot segregate a group of people until you have first done one thing: identified or designated them in terms of at least one criterion that is purportedly relevant in differentiating them from the people who are doing the identifying, designating, differentiating, or segregating. Obviously, this identifying difference must have one very powerful characteristic: it must be seen by the segregators as being very significant.

In truth the one single characteristic of a person, or of a group, that can override *all* other shared characteristics of people in being used as the justification of segregation can be utterly trivial. It is remarkable in itself that one single characteristic can be presumed to differentiate people so totally, i.e., in that this characteristic can override everything else, even thousands of other characteristics that the segregators and the segregatees share. If we just contemplate that one little reality, we may be stunned by its magnitude, especially when we consider that this one overriding characteristic can be something as minor as skin color, the shape of one's ears, left-handedness in Japan, or something of this nature. Even when the characteristic is not trivial, it pales in comparison to the massiveness of the shared characteristics.

Once a group of people are segregated, they are almost invariably congregated. Again, one can cite nursing homes and special classes as examples, as well as almost all the human service agencies that serve devalued people, and that use congregated segregated settings. Congregation reveals one additional belief about segregation: that the congregated, segregated people are not only different from all the rest of the people, but they also *share* some common characteristic(s), and are more like than unlike each other. In a feedback loop, segregatory congregation also signals back to society that the one characteristic that the congregated people supposedly share with each other is more important than all the thousands of characteristics they share with the segregators.

It is a curious phenomenon that distantiation of an unpleasant stimulus object–in our instance, this would be people–is one of the most universal, reflexive, human social responses. It has been so universal across all times, places, and cultures, and so universal even beyond the human species (it is found as a very common response in many animal species) as to suggest that there is some sort of biological function being served by this segregatory impulse.

For this and/or other reasons, if a legitimate overt reason for segregation does not lie close at hand, then totally irrational and infinitely diverse ones will be pressed into service. This strongly suggests that society and people "need" devalued people and groups. If they do not have enough of them, they will manufacture them. They may pick upon almost any characteristic and make that the devalued characteristic on the basis of which segregation can be transacted. Again, that phenomenon is a universal in human experience.

Granted the above, we therefore have to conclude that deviancy-making and segregation are fueled by largely unconscious dynamics, because only through the operation of unconscious dynamics can we manage to focus upon irrelevant and trivial characteristics, and make them the criteria for total, massive, perpetual and "mankind-ever" segregating–which we, as human beings, have always done.

Let us very briefly review a typical sequence in which segregation is acted out, either for an individual or for a group of individuals. We start off with persons who have some characteristic which somehow or other has come to be defined as devalued. Then the person having that characteristic is defined and perceived as socially devalued. The moment that happens, rejection sets in which is one side of the coin, the other side of which is distantiation. Where you find distantiation, you can perforce infer rejection, because when you feel rejection, you will have a nearly irresistible impulse to distantiate. Next, the distantiated and rejected devalued person becomes oppressed, punished, and brutalized, and finally is symbolically "marked" and "branded" as devalued. This symbolic branding takes place through cultural imagery. We have all sorts of polarities of what we consider to be positive and negative. Certain things are valued, and their opposites are devalued. Devalued people get attached with devalued attributes and perceptions. They are seen as old, sick, death-bound, decayed, worthless, dangerous, sinful, etc. These value polarities are translated into symbols and images which are then attached to anything whatsoever that in any way stands for, or is associated with, the devalued group. Thus, the money, the funds, the funders, the funding sources, the funding labels, etc., with which programs for devalued people are financed, tend to get negative imagery and names attached to them. The agencies serving negatively valued people tend to acquire negative images, if they did not already start out as negative agencies for negative people. Coordination and regulatory bodies for services for devalued people tend to be labeled or image-attached with negative symbols, images, and contexts. These image attachments occur all the way down to the physical setting of the facility, its history, the location, what it is close to, how it looks, and whether it is comfortable or not. (Settings for devalued people are almost invariably less beautiful and less comfortable than settings for valued people.) The negative imaging applies also to what devalued people are (directly or indirectly) called, and how they are addressed. The segregation/ congregation also generally tends to take place in a clearly deviancy-branding fashion. For instance, the names of settings and facilities or programs tend to shout out the devalued status of their users. The symbols and images that are attached to the settings or groups, the logos, the designs, the decorations, the furnishings, they all tend to scream out devaluation.

PRE-CHRISTIAN HISTORICAL PATTERNS
OF SEGREGATION/INTEGRATION

Preceding the Christian era, it seems that all of the belief systems that had any impact on the Western world, and perhaps other belief systems as well, have always contained reasons for deviancy-making and segregating. If it was not one reason, it has been another, such as (a) some congenital or adventitious physical characteristic of people (disease, handicaps, age, secondary handicaps, physical features, etc.); (b) people's overt and covert behaviors; or (c) people's descent, nationality, or attributive identity such as caste, or the language they speak, or the ethnic group they derive from.

Perhaps most common as a source of segregation has been ethnicity. Religion, class and caste, contagious disease, and assumed possession by evil spirits have also been prevalent sources. If we look at the history of the Jews, we find them segregating sometimes on the basis of religion itself, or on grounds of ritual cleanliness, or because of their perception of certain people as diseased (maybe having leprosy), or as being possessed by spirits. Sometimes, ethnicity seemed to be a factor. For example, the alien wives were cast out of Israel at the time of the reconstruction of the temple, even if they had embraced the Jewish faith. We also read that to some degree, Jews segregated themselves from each other on the basis of their different languages, since there were synagogues for Jews with different languages. However, some of these segregations were self-elected, and not necessarily imposed–and that makes a critical difference.

HISTORICAL PATTERNS OF SEGREGATION/INTEGRATION
IN THE CHRISTIAN TRADITION

In recent years I developed a deep new interest in the history of human services, especially from early Christian days onward. I have conducted some very extensive research, and believe that there are a number of things which we can now conclude about the stance of Christianity in regard to integration and segregation. One of these is that the early Christians, for hundreds of years, were a very close-knit and self-separatist group–for good reasons. (a) They were a persecuted minority, and therefore had to protect themselves and practice secrecy. (b) Their worship practices were very time-consuming. A great deal of time was spent in prayer, worship and religious fellowship, and after doing all the things involved in daily living, not much time was left for many other kinds of socialization. Consistent with these realities, we have no evidence that Christians segregated themselves from other Christians because of handicap. We do have some evidence to suggest that perhaps they segregated themselves from each other on the basis of language–and, of course, because of various schisms, which started as early as the time of Paul.

The second thing we can conclude is that handicapped and poor people were widely attached with the highest conceivable value because they were seen as the hidden Christ. Hardly ever, in fact, was there any question in Christianity until recently but that any human was fully human. I invite people to search the records of Christian statements on that issue. Handicap was seen as possibly interfering with the soul's operation, the body being the container of the soul; but the soul was believed to be there in its fullness, with its two full attributes of intellect and will merely shackled by an imperfect body. There were only occasional and minor deviations from this belief, to which we should not ascribe a great deal of importance. For example, Luther, together with a lot of other people, believed that the devil could create human shapes without a soul, that these shapes were then nonhuman, and that they did not deserve human treatment. Luther interpreted at least one retarded person this way, but this is a minor aberration which, theologically, was not even far-fetched.[1] So, we should not overplay this minor aberration. In essence, it was a belief in the fullness of the created human that sustained devout Christians everywhere in their belief in the value and the worthiness of intellectually even very incapacitated persons who might not be able to understand the faith, and who might not be able to participate in worship.

Thirdly, human service by early Christians took mostly two forms. One was direct personal giving and helping; the second one was opening one's own home in hospitality to people who were poor, sick, wounded, broken, homeless, or travelers. We have the story of Fabiola, a 4th century Roman matron, who started a hospice in her own home. Another well-known and beloved saint was Saint Elizabeth of Hungary, married to the prince of Thuringia, who made her whole castle over into a hospice for the poor. By definition, this tradition meant that the hospices for the needy, the handicapped, and so on, were the size of somebody's home, that they generally were located where people's homes were located, and that they tended to be highly integrated.

Fourthly, when charity became more organized through the monastic orders, then their chapter houses, settlements, and monasteries (almost every one of the latter) had at least one hospice, a house of hospitality, for wanderers or for anyone in need. Also, these were often attached to churches and especially to cathedrals. Most of these tended to be very small. The classical pattern was a hospice for somewhere between 10 and 14 needy people, in an approximation of the number of apostles (depending on which ones were counted), plus in some cases, Christ. These hospices tended to be very integrated into their monastic or village communities, and this whole pattern persisted until roughly the 1400s.

From earliest time, and throughout the Middle Ages, performing the direct personalistic works of mercy and hospitality were seen as a service to the hidden Christ. "Behold, I stand at the door and knock" (Revelation 3:20). "Who will know that it is me and will administer unto me?" Therefore, the service to the handicapped, to the needy person, the direct, immediate, hands-on service, was seen as one of the most splendid opportunities for Christians to serve upon their Lord, and it was a good fortune to be presented with this opportunity. This is expressed in some quotes. Saint Elizabeth, who gathered up all the afflicted people she could find in the countryside to offer her hospitality to them, said, "How well it is for us that thus we bathe and cover our Lord." Not how good it is for *them*-that is what we say today; but how good it is for *us* that we minister unto the Lord. St. Chrysostomus, the Patriarch of Constantinople (349-407) said, "If there were no poor, the greater part of your sins would not be removed. They are the healers of your wounds" (Thompson & Goldin, 1975, p. 6).

In the same spirit, an abbot said, "Come, draw near to this hospital roof, 0 you travelers overcome by fatigue! Accept the offerings of hospitality, the bread that will nourish your hearts, the good drink flowing freely, clothing to protect you from the cold. These, my friends, are the blessings I, Theognoste, have received from my master Christ, giver of all riches. Thank Him, for it is He who nourishes the world; for me, utter only the prayer that in exchange for this hospitality, I shall be fortunate enough to be taken into the bosom of Abraham" (Thompson & Goldin, 1975, p. 6-7).

Because such a service was a service to and for Christ, and because of the centrality of prayer and worship in a monastery that was properly run, the early hospices were–I found to my amazement–designed as churches. They were constituted of a nave, with an altar at the end, and the beds down the aisle. Initially, there were usually 10-14 beds, all very close to the altar, because mass had to be seen and heard in order to make this service valid, and the facility could therefore not (initially) be very large. That is why the early hospices tended to be called "domus domini" in Latin (house of the Lord); God's house in English; maison Dieu or Hôtel Dieu in French; God-shuizen in Dutch; and so on. Some are called these things to this day, but people no longer know why.

All this also explains why residential facilities in many countries (and in other languages) to this day are called "reception centers," as in Quebec and France. It comes from the French term "Centre d'Accueil." Accuellier in French means to greet, to welcome, to receive, to give ear to. Of course, these centers became our modern institutions with thousands of residents, but they started as centers of welcome, and of voluntary services to the hidden Christ.

These Christian services being voluntary, the hospitality was free. The only requirement was that the recipient pray for the founder. This is why in England, the hospices were called Bedehouses (beden meant to pray).

Around AD 1000, nursing orders started up. In some of them, the members ate cheap bread and used stone utensils, but the "Seigneurs Pauvres" (the Poor Lords) they served on solid silver platters; they served the best wine and meat at least 3 times a week (when hardly anyone else in those days was getting it); they gave them a fur cap, fur coat, and fur shoes so that they could get up out of bed in comfort when they had to–and all of this was free.

By 436 AD, the Council of Carthage specifically urged the bishops to maintain hospices "in close proximity to churches." (That is exactly the way it says in the Latin. Some of these things are so unbelievable that I went back to the original Latin just to make sure that the translations had not lost some of the meaning, but I found that some of the Latin was even stronger than some of the translations.) This edict of the Council was followed all over Christendom. The bishops started hospices, and these were generally literally "in the shadow" of the cathedrals.

Our history books tell us that residential institutions (for the mentally disordered, retarded, etc.) are relatively new, with beginnings in the 18th and 19th century. I was amazed to find that human services history is taught in a way that distorts the facts, and denies the continuity of all sorts of developments. In fact, medieval Europe was covered with thousands upon thousands of hospices–and all together, these helping forms were highly integrated. They were in the shadow of the centrally placed town church to begin with; they were in the hustling, bustling monasteries, many of which, in those days, were not at all in quiet, far-off places; they were in the middle of villages and towns; they were in people's houses within the villages and towns. By church law, retarded people, specifically, were to be baptized, and the law encouraged their church attendance and even communion–which later on we forgot about. (But, of course, for a long time, even most non-retarded people communicated only once a year.) The law or its interpreters even encouraged confirmation (Pickett, 1952), although this was not always practiced.

The fifth major point we can bring out is that all sorts of segregatory practices also prevailed in Christian Europe, but that these largely involved caste and class, rather than handicap. By and large, these types of segregation were not even of such a nature that made it unlikely for a member of the more valued classes to be totally unfamiliar with the lives of the less valued classes. Also, at least theologically, there was no argument but that before God, people were indeed equal. Until about the 1500s, apparently the only truly outcast groups were "the infidel" and people with leprosy, and lepers might even be permitted to remain in their houses or live on the edge of town.

Systematic segregation and brutalization came in with the rise of intellect, rationality, science, empiricism, learning, the Renaissance, and so on. This emphasis upon worldly accomplishment was also somewhat facilitated by the trends associated with the Reformation. The Reformation also indirectly contributed to the plight of the handicapped, in two ways. One was that it eliminated several thousand hospices that were run by religious orders, because the orders themselves were eliminated. When the orders were eliminated, you had a problem, namely the people who served in the hospices had made vows of celibacy and poverty. When you lift the vows of celibacy and poverty, then you get what you have today: people get married, have their own families to attend to, and will or can no longer voluntarily, in poverty, serve upon the handicapped. As a result, there was a practically total collapse of the hospice system in Protestant northern Europe. In turn, that contributed secondarily or tertiarily to yet other problematic service developments. Since the celibate poverty-bound servant had vanished, people started charitable foundations with hired employees. I propose that that was the beginning of the human service worker of today–a paid hireling who serves as a career because s/he gets paid for it, instead of doing it voluntarily, in poverty, as a life vocation. This development contributed to what we might call the commercialization of human services, which is a third-order derivative, but it undermined the perception of the needy person as a precious member of the wounded body of Christ.

Really large-scale segregation and congregation commenced when contagious diseases and epidemics broke out, particularly in the 1600s and 1700s. At the same time, the criminalization of poverty also took place. Elizabethan poor laws made poverty almost a crime. In France, Louis XIV issued edicts in 1656 for the building of huge institutions to congregate all the unwanted people of society, and get them out of the way.

In another sudden surge of scientism in the late 1840s, segregation became systematized via large-scale agency founding. We interpret this as a period of reform and positive measures, but the fact is that these foundations were professionalistic and agencyistic, staffed by paid career human service workers. The service foundations of the Reformation era became thus translated into modernism.

The bottom fell out of human service morality in any number of ways when medicine unequivocally abandoned its moral, philosophical, and theological background, abandoned "moral treatment" (an enlightened method prevalent between about 1800-1850), and fully and unequivocally embraced materialistic science as its religion. This happened roughly between 1870 and 1890–a relatively short time span. Fittingly, this development was tied in with the onset of genetics, social Darwinism, and the genetic alarm. Of course, medicine was not alone, but it served as the major spearhead in the application of materialistic science to human service, and largely dragged with it the early equivalents of social work, psychology, rehabilitation, and in some degree even education.

Materialistic medicine (and its allies) hit one of its peaks between 1920 and 1945. In 1920, an infamous little book was written (Binding and Hoche) which was later adopted by the Nazis, and which was the first modern succinct and total justification for euthanasia. Its fruit was the mass destruction of handicapped people and other devalued groups during World War II. The excesses of materialistic medicine were so shocking to the world that after 1945, that particular ideology went partially underground, but it is now reemerging in full force, and is moving once more to the destruction of those people who are perceived as seriously and "incurably" impaired or diseased –which, of course, includes the moderately, severely and profoundly retarded.

Now it is essential to be deeply aware of such secular trends, because any major or enduring secular trend will find an expression in the church. If we have a glorification of technology in society, then even in the churches, we will see technology elevated. We may see it in the technologization of religious instruction; in pastors calling upon scientists, psychologists, counselors and therapists–upon secular science, so to speak–to solve age-old problems of suffering; etc. If we see dehumanization in the culture, then we will see it in the churches, such as we saw in the 1977 Task Force on Human Life report of the Anglican Church in Canada that came out and explained why and how Christianity tells us that retarded people are not human and should not live. The imprint of Christianity will be put upon all sorts of evil things–which is why we see segregation practiced on a massive scale in practically all denominations, and why other secular and even idolatrous practices are widely recapitulated in the churches without being labeled as such, and often without being recognized. Given Satan's strategies, that is what we should expect: secular practices, and even idolatrous ones, as when what is called (in several languages) the carer of souls (the word for minister or priest) calls upon the scientist to save a person from the human condition.

JUDEO-CHRISTIAN RATIONALES FOR INTEGRATION

We now review some Judeo-Christian rationales for integration, and combine these with an appeal to an integrative-liberating approach.

While I was preparing this paper, I mused just what one might draw upon in one's analysis and search for rationales for integration or segregation of one group of people by another. It occurred to me that there might be six major sources of analysis: (a) divine laws and commandments; (b) general principles of Christian moral theology; (c) the precedents set by Christ; (d) inference of what Christ would likely have done had He come in this time and world; (e) the examples set by the lives of great saints; and (f) divine guidance and revelation in the here and now.

Divine Laws and Commandments

One source might be to examine divine laws and commandments to see what, if anything, there is which bears on what we now call integration or segregation. Here, we must not rule out the possibility that even the mass practices of entire churches may be in violation of divine law. The very fact that the mass practices of Christian churches today is almost diametrically opposed to the mass practices of the early and even medieval church tells us that one of the two patterns must be wrong, or that there is nothing in divine law that has a bearing on the issue of integration/segregation–which is difficult to believe. If there is relevant law, then it should be followed regardless of prevailing practices.

If we look at the law, we would have to stretch the ten commandments if we are to find anything to support segregation. One can point to certain passages and implications of the law as making segregating defensible, but one would still have to stretch it. However, one does not have to stretch the law to find rationales in support of integration. For example, if we look at the command to love one's neighbor, together with the hypocrite, we may ask, "and who is my neighbor"? Does it include the retarded, disordered, elderly, prisoner, law offender, poor, racial minority member, foreigner, etc.? Next, can we not safely assume that in order to love one's neighbor, the neighbor first would presumably have to be somewhere around to be loved? If the neighbor is nowhere near, is far away, or is segregated and congregated, it makes hollow that particular command. Also, loving one's neighbor seems to imply that the neighbor should probably enjoy the same benefits and privileges that I enjoy, and should be no more restricted than I myself would like to be restricted.

Also of relevance to integration may be the fourth commandment to honor one's parents. Can this law be considered met by the wholesale congregation of elderly people in segregated housing–even if such housing were benign rather than vicious, or corrupt? Does the fact that churches sponsor housing and other programs for the elderly meet the command if the elderly people are distinctly, unnecessarily, and to a significant degree against their will segregated from society?

Is the proven fact that discontinuity in abode and relationships tends to hasten the deaths of vulnerable people not relevant to the law that says, "thou shalt not kill"?

Many patterns of segregation require that people divest themselves of their individual belongings. Has this no bearing on the law against stealing? And is it not true that the preservation of individual belongings is one of the perennial and almost insuperable problems of segregated residential settings of even moderate size?

When we exaggerate the importance of relatively trivial attributes of people by using these attributes as justifications for segregation, are we not bearing false witness against that which defines these people (now devalued) as our brothers and sisters?

What about the many positive commands (especially in the Old Testament, such as Isaiah) to befriend and defend the weak and helpless, to correct aggression, to procure justice, etc.–are these commandments met by assuring that "we" as well as other people have minimal personal contact with devalued people? Are we protecting endangered people from *our* aggression by segregating them away?

General Principles of Christian Moral Theology

Furthermore, beyond the clear-cut divine laws and commandments, there are general principles of Christian moral theology which are inferred from divine laws, commandments, precepts and so on. One very relevant principle here is that behavior that might be morally defensible is not necessarily optimal. This type of rule is commonly encountered in moral theology. For instance, striving for sanctity means that one does more than the minimum necessary for salvation, and every person should strive for sanctity, within their strength. Another example is that one might be morally justified in resisting an aggressor, but just about everybody would agree that pacifism, non-violence and offering the other cheek is infinitely more in the Christian ideal than justified resistance. To our issue, that means that even where there might be reasons that might justify imposed segregation, e.g., perhaps of people who are interpreted as a nuisance or even as a danger, then even more Christian would be to forbear, to risk, to carry a burden, and to accept any suffering which that might entail.

The Precedents Set by Christ

A third very major source of guidance would be to examine Christ's life. What did Christ do? It always amazes me that our churches do not ask that when they deal with impaired people. Whom did Christ segregate, and whom did He integrate? What is the evidence?

Perhaps the most segregated group of people in Biblical times were those with leprosy. Christ went far beyond curing any leprous person that asked for help. He did what not even the family members of a person with leprosy would do. Here is a retelling of the story (Donders, 1978). "A man crawled up to Jesus on his knees, with his clothing torn and his hair disordered, shielding his upper lip with his right hand, shouting, 'unclean, unclean,' all according to the prescriptions of the old, old testament. But between those words imposed on him by religious law, he whispered, 'if you want to, you can cure me,' and (Jesus) said, 'of course I want to,' *and he touched him.*"

You have got to appreciate leprosy and the law: you never touched the leprous person who was the most outcast, untouchable creature under heaven. But Christ touched the man with leprosy.

Another outcast class were prostitutes and adulteresses. Christ had himself washed and anointed by one; and in fact, he seemed to have a very special concern for them. He showed a tender mercy for the woman taken only minutes before in the very act of adultery.

Tax collectors had betrayed the anointed nation and had sold their services to a pagan idolatrous conqueror. Christ feasted with them congenially, while at the feasts of the rich and of the powerful, he brought embarrassment.

Another deeply devalued group were the Samaritans who were seen as worse than pagans because they were perceived as apostate and/or racially defiled Jews. But Christ interacted with them, accepted ritually polluted drink from a Samaritan woman, and held up the Good Samaritan as an example of God-fearing charity. He not only healed the Gerasene outcast who had evil spirits, but sat with him afterwards.

In a culture dominated by males and by elders, he bent over backward in according status to women. For instance, the remarkable fact that after his resurrection, he appeared to the women first, and especially to Mary Magdalene, appears to be grossly underinterpreted in its significance. Even in death, Christ chose to hang with two criminals, one who rejected him, and one who accepted him.

Did Christ impose segregation on any group? From Scripture, we cannot conclude that he did. The closest thing he did to segregrating was to chase the merchants out of the temple, and that is not really a sufficient enough analogy for what we usually mean by segregation. In fact, as one writer put it in his book, Christ spent a great deal of his time in pretty bad company (*Jesus in Bad Company*, Holl, 1971). So we must perforce conclude that our segregating practices have no precedent in Christ's life.

Inference of What Christ Would Likely Have Done Had He Come in This Time and World

This then leads us to the next question; and again, it is a remarkable question which churches do not seem to address very well today. It is very simple: let us assume that Christ had not come 2,000 years ago, but that He had come for His mission today, in this age, and this culture. There are some reasonably strong inferences that we can draw as to what Christ would have done today. Can anyone seriously propose that Christ would have told us that we should build institutions for the retarded, for the mentally disordered, or the elderly? If Christ were to come today, he would probably spend many of his nights, and take many of his meals, in our racial city ghettoes, and that is probably where he would perform a great deal of his preaching and healing. He would almost certainly have visited some of our segregated programs and institutions. He would have confounded the wisdom of the scientists and of the professionals by his deeds there. While he would have cured the people with epilepsy, venereal diseases, cerebral palsy, mental disorder and even mental retardation, to keepers of the many miserable human service settings, he would probably have said, "Let go my people; liberate the captives; and you yourselves go and sin no more."

The Examples Set by the Lives of the Great Saints

The next source is the examples set in and by the lives of the great saints. The lives of the great saints are not, and cannot be expected to be, as clear-cut, consistent, and perfect as that of Christ. However, one hallmark and major characteristic of the saints has always been the opening of doors, peacemaking, uniting, bringing people together, reconciling, sharing, and living with–these are often the very things that cause us to say that someone is a saint when we see him/her doing these things. Some saints have started services which ended up segregated, and even perverted, but rarely did they become fully segregated and perverted until the saint's successors took over. So the lives of the saints are much more consistent with integrative life-sharing than are patterns of service that increase the likelihood of devalued people being cut off from society.

Divine Guidance and Revelation in the Here and Now

I now come to a most peculiar category of seeking the guidance and the revelation of the Spirit in the here and now. When I make a presentation, I can often sense when I am coming to a point where there is going to be a misinterpretation of what I say; this is one of those moments. By seeking divine guidance and revelation, I am referring to a process in which we consciously, with full awareness of what we are doing, address the issue of integration/segregation over an extended period of time, and in committed seeking and searching in the fellowship of a community of faithful people who, in community, join in a willingness and preparedness to surrender their own egos, their desires, and their technologies; and who are willing to do what the Spirit may tell them. Thus, a community of the faithful who desire divine guidance should enter this process in earnest prayer and petition, communally, and publicly. By publicly, I mean not each person quietly praying, but by stating verbally their petitions for guidance, their surrender to the Spirit. They must do it as a community over time, and be willing to accept the answer when it comes, and not stick to the predisposed solutions that they may have come with. There are thus six elements here: consciousness, earnestness, extended time to permit the Spirit to descend and speak, fellowship, petitions, and a public communal nature of petitioning.[2]

We almost never do this sort of discerning. Entire groups and service communities have started service patterns without doing this. We should not be surprised about the perversions that happen not just 100 or 500 years later, but within 5 years, or even one year, because such developments are built on the ego, on technology, and not on the Spirit. Yet when we do these six things, it would appear to me that Scripture has told us that we will be told what to do. "I shall be with you until the end of days." The Spirit will be sent, and on and on. The promise is unequivocally there. The answer that we may get when it comes to an issue of integration or segregation may come in unexpected ways, and may not always be what we, at this moment, and in a normalization sense, may interpret to be integration; but one thing it will certainly then be: an answer that will bring an opening of people, a proliferation of vocations to life-sharing, etc. In that sense, at the very least, there will be integration; and perhaps often, it will be integration in the usual sense.

IMPLICATIONS FOR THE BEHAVIOR OF INTEGRATORS

A review of these six guides thus comes down very heavily on the side of integration but we have not yet spelled out all the rationales that may underline these principles as they bear on a potential integrator's behavior. Such rationales might include the following:

1. There has always been the implication in Christian tradition that it is justified, and sometimes called for, to work out one's salvation in the midst of the world's suffering. Not everybody needs to be everywhere, but always where there is suffering, some people are called to be present, to work out their salvation by sharing, and thus to bear witness to God's glory and power. This means that many integrators must "report for duty" where the suffering is explicitly present.

2. We are called to genuinely share the lives and the suffering of devalued people, especially the very way that Christ did by example. By example, he did it, not just with the specially devalued people, but he shared the suffering of the humanness of all humanity in general. He took all this upon himself, and shared it, but He did share especially with the poor and the rejected.

3. By extending oneself into integration, especially via life-sharing, one expresses one's solidarity with a group that is devalued or oppressed, and one rejects or refuses to act out the devaluing segregation imposed by others. In that sense, one imitates Christ, and *imitatio Christi* is an old tradition within the church. Indeed, the segregation that is often imposed or glorified by the

world should not merely be rejected by Christian allies of the devalued, but should be *confronted* both by the word and in prophetic action, and what better way to accomplish this than in the Christian churches, worship, and instruction.

4. Yet another implication is that by extending oneself to the devalued people, one thereby gets closer to the transaction of the ministry to the needy–to those in need of food, shelter, clothes, consolation, encouragement, and so on. Again, one does not accomplish this by segregating oneself, or the needy.

5. Relatedly, in service to the needy, one serves upon the wounded body of Christ. Remember the corporal works of mercy: the person in need, the devalued, the oppressed, and typically the segregated people, they are the hidden Christ waiting to be recognized and served upon; they are the crucified body of Christ–even more crucified than other people.

6. Finally, one exerts positive influence on non-believers and sinners by modeling and preaching. It is very hard to evangelize if one does not do at least a little bit of modeling.

Insofar as many devalued people represent the hidden Christ waiting to be recognized and admitted, the unnecessary segregation of such people is not only theologically unsound, but may actually represent a Satanic strategy, thereby constituting patterned evil. It is no coincidence that successful rites of exorcism such as practiced by some African communities (cited in Montgomery, 1973, P. 181 ff.) are also rites of social (re)integration, in which the participation of the community of the faithful is essential, with the expectation that the possessed person, once cleansed, will be part of that community.

If one perceives the Satanic urgency in the reflexiveness of segregation, one can also become much clearer in one's own mind why institutional segregation of the mentally retarded, the mentally disordered, and many other handicapped groups has never really "worked," at least over the long run and as a patterned policy. Inevitably, and apparently *everywhere* in the world, it has eventually resulted in profound and systematic evil and abuses, and must be expected to do the same in the future. Over time, even institutions founded with the noblest of purposes inevitably attract evil like a magnet, in a pattern which has such timeless universality that it is phenomenal that it is recognized by so few people as being a genuine and overriding universal. Again, the empirical facts are so compelling that only Satanic deception can account for their widespread rejection. Thus, a sound perspective on the patterning of evil in human services and service structures can yield most valuable insights of an extremely practical nature as regards specific service provisions and patterns. However, it must not be assumed that the identification and elimination of one patterning of evil will automatically result in the elimination of the imposition of evil practices upon a devalued group. It is quite to be expected that one evil pattern will merely be succeeded by another. Yet, this reality in no way diminishes one's responsibility to stand up against *any* of the evil patterns. It is fully to be expected that the hidden Christ will always attract Satanic persecution and deception, and our challenge is to strive to recognize its expression in all of its forms.

ARE THERE ANY RATIONALES FOR SEGREGATION?

Having looked into integration, what then might be some plausible valid rationales within Christianity for segregation? One could say that some persons or groups make the lives of others unmanageable, i.e., offend against society so greatly that other people cannot carry out their lives, and therefore some form of segregation may need to be effectuated. Perhaps there are people who have chosen to commit sins which other people simply cannot abide, i.e., the presence of a certain type of sinfulness may not be manageable for others, perhaps by constituting excessive temptation. All this is quite conceivable, and these rationales might therefore be valid. However, these rationales may not be valid for segregating a specific offending person; they may be more valid for removing oneself. Thus, one might try to keep from falling into temptation and corruption by seeking environments and people that are apart from the ones that are engaging in patterns and sins which I find too much to bear. I may want to remove myself, I may want to protect my family, my children from certain influences, etc., but this is not to be confused with imposed segregation on a societally devalued and less powerful group. In fact, it may be the other way around. It may be the powerful majority that may be doing these things from which I might have to remove myself.

Another argument that might be presented even from a Christian perspective is that by segregating, one might be able to teach or habilitate devalued people or groups more effectively. There are three things to consider when this argument is presented: (a) As such segregation is so often practiced within the churches, the rationale is usually not valid. It is a secular, technological, scientific argument that says that the secular pedagogic technologies will be more effective than the Christian sharing. Yet, we know as a fact that the argument is usually untrue, *even* on the technical level. One usually does not teach and habilitate better by segregating people into congregated, segregated, deviancy cultures. (b) Secondly, we know that in fact, the segregated people not only usually learn less, but that additionally, over the long run, this type of segregation results in people remaining, or becoming even more, devalued–if not this group of people, then the vast number of people who are devalued for the same reason. Revaluation of people is not readily achieved in isolation; there are usually generalization effects in operation. (c) Thirdly, the argument is purely technical, not a theological one, and theological issues must take precedence over any issue of technology. Even if it were true that segregation brings better teaching and habilitation, first comes the kingdom of God, and its precepts and demands. If people are going to be less bright, less skilled, etc., within the kingdom, then so be it. Bodily, social and technological achievement is not the ultimate calling of human beings.

One area in which our churches commonly segregate is in the religious education of handicapped people. There may well be a very valid reason for some such segregation, but it would seem that validity would only follow if we have examined the following issues:

First, were we totally unable to think of any other alternatives that would have been more integrated? Did we even try to have another alternative? Was there a sincere attempt to find an alternative that was adequately supported? Was it an attempt by people who wanted it to succeed? We have a huge number of religious empires in North America, some of them are very well known, that are aimed at handicapped people. They are really idolatrous; power-hungry clergy are often in charge; there was never any intent or desire to integrate in the first place before the segregated empire was started. Yet, even technology and science could come to our aid, because we know what some of the technologies are that help people integrate. Even though a lot of this technology is available, we have rarely even attempted to integrate. How many options did we give a chance before we segregated? If we did not try to integrate, and/or still have untried options, then I would say that any segregation we structure is, in itself, unacceptable and in violation of our precepts.

I find it almost impossible to conceive of a situation where integration would fail if it were sought and conducted in commitment to the Spirit. Such a failure would probably tell us that the particular congregation or setting is no longer a religious one, but one masquerading as such–though quite likely unconsciously. However, let us assume we had done everything we could, and some form of segregation still seemed to be indicated, we must then ask if it is the minimal segregation consistent with fulfilling its purpose–no more than is absolutely necessary. The larger the number of devalued people that one congregates, the more barriers against the outside one sets up. Is the congregating which we do the minimal, the smallest, congregating that is necessary in this instance? Is the segregation and the congregating minimally deviancy-imaged and maximally value-imaged? Quite often, deviancy-imaging is epidemic.

Have we, furthermore, bent over backward suspecting our own motives? Segregation is fueled by universal unconscious dynamics, so we have to assume that not one of us is fully conscious of the dynamics of his/her desires or devaluations. Have I suspected my motives, or are we going around and glorifying the segregation–as we often do?

And finally, again, did we urgently pray for another alternative? Was there a sincere petition on the issue *before* we started? Did we pray for integrative supports and integrative supporters, for assimilators to step forward? Did we bring our hopes and prayers to the congregation as a whole? Did we even go to the church, to the congregation, and say, here are rejected people, what can we do? Let the Spirit come and guide us. Did we interpret the issues to the congregation in the light of Scriptures? Did we go and preach from the pulpit what the Scriptures and the life of Christ say? Did we act in faith? Did we surrender to the Spirit, or did we treat segregation as an egotistical technology, as an extension of a lack of faith, or as a faith in technology rather than in the Spirit and the promise? Utilization of all these conceivable measures is almost unheard of.

Perhaps the most common rationale that appears to be advanced on behalf of segregation by religious people is that it serves for the protection of the segregated groups from harm, or from greater harm. That is probably the most difficult argument to deal with, because it contains some truth, some unconscious attribution of one's own rejection to others, some non-truth, some myth. The fact is that when you segregate a sub-group of a devalued class of people, you contribute to the long-term systemic devaluation of the entire class, which leads to yet greater needs for protection from danger in the future. Furthermore, we know that when devalued people are segregated and congregated, we create patterns of desensitization of the public, and mentalities that tend toward violence. Again, how many thousands of years of history do we need to see the obvious here? In time, violence typically even comes from the service workers themselves, and not just from other people. In almost every segregated service system for devalued people which human beings have ever created, the service workers eventually have transacted violence toward the people they served. Also, even if it were true that one might protect an endangered group by segregation, even then it might not be desirable or sound to offer that special protection, because we are all called to suffering, and the prevention of one evil must not be achieved at the price of contributing to an even greater evil. At least in the Christian theology, the inevitability of suffering is in the essence of the faith. Thus, to *disproportionately* try to prevent the suffering of one group may be denying the reality, truth, and purpose of suffering in general.

One related argument that might be heard is that certain segregated service patterns are more apt to enable a person to practice the faith. For instance, it might be legitimate for a church to establish a housing project designed to enable people of faith to practice it intently by being close to a chapel, by special scheduling of the prayer routine, by having ministers at hand, by banning certain sinful customs within the project, or things of this nature. But by what rationale could a church-affiliated project go the next step and, say, ban children, or ban middle-aged adults from living there, or permit only handicapped people to live there and to practice their faith–yet that is what our projects so often do. Or what if we started such a project, but structured it in such a fashion that nobody who is not a member of a societally devalued class would freely choose to be there, to be part of it, or live there? This we also do so often when the service settings are so structured that nobody would choose to be there, or live there, if they were not forced to do so by circumstances.

By what Christian rationale can our churches justify the congregating of people who are devalued by society in such huge numbers that the very fact of their large congregation calls for the employment of hirelings to come in 37.5 hours a week to do something or other, sometimes even something that might not have been needed had the congregating not been so big? Indeed, let us go one step further! What is implied if one started out with the prevailing rationales in the churches, regarding special housing and whatever, and then did not even follow through and honor the sustenance of the religious atmosphere? This might happen if one admitted people to the special setting who rejected the religious assumptions and the religious life that the church presumably tried to create. What if church-affiliated settings employed hirelings who reject the faith and its practices–which is exactly what our churches of all major denominations are doing today in order to get public money, that ancient idol god. Why do we need public monies to run a service that ends up not living up to our faith, *and* that is segregated and congregated? Does not that kind of money-grabbing and service-running become idolatrous, or at the very least faithless? Is it not a throwing away of good money (donated by the faithful) after bad (public money used faithlessly)?

So, again, the rationales in support of integration seem to greatly outweigh just about any of the rationales that we might put forth on a Christian basis on behalf of segregation. All of that raises agonizing challenges to the systematically practiced segregation in and by the churches that we see everywhere we look, in practically all the denominations. Some of the things that we see being used to combat this are very beautiful; but by and large, the major pattern is that of segregation in all sorts of means and ways by churches and by Christians. Even if they do not practice segregation outright, the feebleness with which the message and theology of integration is preached and taught within the churches increases the challenge.

Especially when people are segregated essentially against their will, when they have no meaningful choice and/or alternatives, and when that kind of segregation is interpreted as being for their own good, then I would be inclined to say that the most plausible thing to do is to start off by suspecting Satanic deception. Much as moral theologians have always preached that one should not only refrain from sin but one should in addition avoid the occasion for sin (where the circumstance and the setting for the likelihood of one's sinning is increased), so should devout people bend over backward in suspecting the legitimacy of segregation, and seek vigorously for a means of doing all the good things we say we want to do–in an integrated fashion.

CONCLUDING REFLECTION

Neither the Jewish nor the Christian faith is quite rational–nor were they meant to be. The greatness of God transcends all our feeble human intelligence, even though the human intellect is made in the likeness and image of God. The Christian faith is even less rational than the Jewish faith, and the fact that the Christian God incarnated as a suffering God can ultimately only be accepted; it really cannot be understood, no matter what our educated theologians may say about it. It is from this mystery that many other mysteries flow, including, and especially relevant to us, God's special compassion for the littlest people, and the suffering; and that it is especially through suffering people that the suffering God of Christianity manifests Himself. Especially the wounds that are inflicted by power, wealth, strength, health, etc., on littler people have always been likened to the wounds of Christ. Christ died for our sins; and not just for our past sins, but also for future sins. It is in this sense that brutalities or injustices that are inflicted recapitulate the crucifixion endlessly; and in turn, the crucifixion endlessly recapitulates for every sinner the possibility and the promise, if the sinner so chooses, of salvation.

Now this is why the crucifixion must be made known and public. Christ was lifted up on a tree for all to see, as Moses lifted up the serpent, so that sinners might see the suffering of God's holy one, repent, believe, and be saved. The crucifixions of devalued people, in and out of human services, must not be hidden. They must not be shipped out and away and put behind the doors, behind the gates, and into the towers. Those crucifixions must be as public and visible and as lifted up, as was Christ himself. How did doubting Thomas come to believe? He put his fingers into Christ's open wound, and when he was able to touch the wound, it was then that he was able to say, "My Lord, my *God!*"

The incarnate Christ has ascended, but he has left us the wounds to touch. The wounds are, especially, the suffering of the disadvantaged, or even oppressed. They are the ones who are recrucified perpetually, and so there is a perpetual wound, and they are the specially wounded members of Christ's body. It is these wounded members of Christ's body that we must touch, because like Thomas, it is by reverently touching them that our faith is strengthened. So this facsimile of Christ is not to be hidden, is not to be locked up or removed from the presence of society or from the naves of the churches. It is not to be disguised, reinterpreted, or what have you. The wounds have to be there for all to see, and have to be lifted up in the market place, by the gate, at the doors of the temple, or wherever people naturally gather. Then people can choose whether they want to repent, believe, serve, accept, or reject. And we, as Christian human service workers, will serve doubly by bringing together the suffering Christ with the potential or actual believer. The potential believer is infinitely more apt to become a real believer who will try to extend justice and compassion to a wounded person; and the wounded person is thereby vastly more likely to be healed from the wounds of oppression–and it is in these double healings that God is glorified.

NOTES

1. To this day, some theologians believe it is possible that demons can take on human shape (e.g., Montgomery, 1976).
2. This is not to deny the need for and efficacy of private approaches as well, but it appears that the weight of the promise of divine guidance lies with communality.

REFERENCES

Binding, K., and Hoche, A. (1920) *Die Friegabe der vernichtung Lebensunwerten Lebens: Ihr Mass und ihre Form.* Leipzig, Germany: Felix Meiner.

Donders, J. (1978) Sins are the trouble. In J.G. Donders, *Jesus the stranger.* Maryknoll, N.Y.: Orbis Books.

Holl, A. (1971) *Jesus in bad company.* (S. King, trans.) New York: Holt, Rinehart and Winston (Originally published in German by Deutsche Verlags-Anstalt, Stuttgart).

Montgomery, J. (1976) (Ed.) *Demon possession: A medical, historical, theological, and anthropological symposium.* Minneapolis, MN: Bethany Fellowship.

Pickett, R.D. (1952) *Mental affliction and church law.* Ottawa, ON: University of Ottawa Press.

Stringfellow, W. (1973) *An ethic for Christians and other aliens in a strange land.* Waco, TX: Word Books.

Thompson, J.D., and Goldin, G. (1975) *The hospital: A social and architectural history.* New Haven, CT: Yale University Press.

An Attempt to Gain a Better Understanding from a Christian Perspective of What "Mental Retardation" Is

Wolf Wolfensberger, PhD

What follows below is an attempt to gain a better understanding of what "mental retardation" is, based on a Christian perspective and on a few assumptions and beliefs that have deep roots and a long tradition in Christianity.

SOME TRADITIONAL CHRISTIAN BASELINE BELIEFS OR TEACHINGS ABOUT HUMAN NATURE

To begin with, and before examining "mental retardation" specifically, I will present seven traditional and widely accepted Christian beliefs, assumptions or propositions about the nature of human beings.

1. Human souls are spirits. Angels are also spirits, but unlike angels, human souls were meant to be united to material bodies.
2. Spirits have intellect and will. In the case of human souls, these have long been called the "faculties" of the soul.
3. There is no reason to assume that all spirits are created alike. Indeed, there is every indication that God has endowed spirits differentially. Ergo, some souls may differ in the degree of intellect that they possess. However, it is much more difficult to conceive of differences in "strength of will" among spirits.
4. In its intended "extra-fallen" state, i.e., in its pre-fallen state, as well as in its future resurrected state after Christ's restoration of creation, the

Reprinted with permission from *National Apostolate with Mentally Retarded Persons Quarterly*, 1982, *13*(3), 2-7.

[Haworth co-indexing entry note]: "An Attempt to Gain a Better Understanding from a Christian Perspective of What 'Mental Retardation' Is." Wolfensberger, Wolf. Co-published simultaneously in *Journal of Religion, Disability & Health* (The Haworth Pastoral Press, an imprint of The Haworth Press, Inc.) Vol. 4, No. 2/3, 2001, pp. 71-83; and: *The Theological Voice of Wolf Wolfensberger* (ed: William C. Gaventa, and David L. Coulter) The Haworth Pastoral Press, an imprint of The Haworth Press, Inc., 2001, pp. 71-83.

soul is united with a body–indeed, possibly even with its very own, specific and unique, body.

5. However, in its extra-fallen state, the human body is radically different from the fallen body we know. The intended body exists of, and in, a state of matter that obeys an entirely different set of laws (which one might call "physical" only by analogy, hence the quotation marks) than the body we know within our fallen estate.

6. Within the fallen estate, the human soul must be considered multiply hindered. It is hindered by its own fallenness and alienation from God, by the fallenness (and hence imperfection) of the body, and by the imperfection of the union of body and soul. Even within these constraints, the soul's functioning is further hindered by the fact that probably no, or only few, humans ever lived in whom even the natural (fallen) combination of all elements of the body were as unimpeded as they might theoretically be even within their fallen estate.

7. In the extra-fallen state, the soul is not impeded in its functioning by the fall and by the imperfections of a fallen body. Thus, the soul will express itself fully in the extra-fallen domain.

IMPLICATIONS OF THE BASELINE BELIEFS OR TEACHINGS TO OUR UNDERSTANDING OF MENTAL RETARDATION

Given the above, we can make a number of statements as to how mental retardation can be viewed from a traditional Christian perspective.

1. Obviously, any number of limitations and afflictions of the body can impede a person in exercising one or all of the faculties of its soul; and such impediments can range in degree from mild to possibly total.

2. Various impediments imposed by the fallen body upon the fallen soul will be characterized in various ways by our fallen human perception and language.

3. A number of patterns of impediment, even uneven patterns of impairment of the soul's faculties, may end up being called "mental retardation" in our fallen human way of characterizing our experiences–as long as the pattern includes sufficient types and degrees of impairment of intellect. This is apparent from the fact that people with very dissimilar psychometric profiles may be "identified" ("diagnosed") as being mentally retarded, including people with considerable competence, and with a wide range of impairments of volition.

4. On the basis of the traditional Christian belief that God endows his created spirits (angels and souls) with different amounts of intellect, one might even argue that a person (within the fallen domain) could be retarded even if there were no significant bodily imperfections other than those im-

plied by the fall generally. In other words, persons of perfectly healthy bodies might vary widely in their intellects, and even in their personalities, regardless of similar (or even identical) life experiences. However, because spirits are naturally capable of functioning at a high level of abstraction, it is extremely unlikely that any created spirit would be so poorly intellectually endowed as to be viewed by humans as "mentally retarded." In other words, what humans call mental retardation must, most likely, be viewed as entirely a manifestation of an impaired body rather than of the poor endowment of a soul's intellect.

5. The difference between retarded and non-retarded people is infinitesimal as compared to the difference between the fallen and the extra-fallen human estate. The latter difference is so gross as to be inexpressible in fallen human language–and with the exception of rare instances of fall–transcendence, all human communication involves fallen language.

6. Insofar as the soul's expression of its intellect can be impeded by bodily imperfections, we must fully expect that bodily impairment will also often impede the exercise of the other faculty of the soul, i.e., the will.

7. Volition probably plays a major role in phenomena such as suggestibility, how easily one is led astray, whether one can form deep and lasting love relationships, how strongly one can and will commit oneself to a cause or faith, etc. Indeed, in such things, retarded people are commonly weak. For instance, their love relationships are often superficial, less enduring unless materially and appetitively reinforced, and more easily undermined by selfishness or distractions (including competing appetites and reinforcements); their judgments (as verified by many experiments) are very unstable and can easily be swayed–so much that it might be made to swing from one extreme to another (poor judgment must here be distinguished from unstable judgment); etc.

8. The more deeply the exercise of the intellect is impeded, (a) the more greatly we can assume the body to be impaired, regardless of whether this impairment is as yet identifiable; and (b) the greater is the likelihood (at least on a purely probabilistic basis, i.e., across random groups of persons) that the exercise of the will is impaired as well. Indeed, the more deeply the intellect is impaired, the more deleterious is apt to be a negative feedback loop in which intellectual impairment leads to poor bodily competence, body care, self-protection, etc.; and thus, additional bodily damage is apt to result which can even further impede both intellect and will. The presence and strength of this negative feedback cycle must be expected to be linked to how early in life bodily imperfections exist, and for how long they interfere with intellectual development.

It is interesting that the materialistic psychology and education of the modernistic world have largely failed to perceive the frequency, extent and importance of the volitional deficit in retarded people. This deficit is virtually unmentioned (at least not explicitly) in the major formal scientific-profes- sional definitions of mental retardation of the twentieth century. One of the partial exceptions to this reality might be the concept of intelligence held by David Wechsler (author of the various Wechsler intelligence scales) who saw intellect as inseparable from "personality."

In contrast to this inability or reluctance of modern materialistic psycholo- gy to tie intellect and will together, Edouard Seguin (1812-1880, a pioneer in the moral treatment of retarded persons, and in services to retarded people in France and the United States) went even further than the view expressed here, and postulated that volitional impairment was an essential element of mental retardation.

9. It is an empirical observation rather than a conclusion that could be readily reached from (Christian) theology that impairment of intellect with- out concomitant impairment of volition is much rarer than is impairment of volition without concomitant impairment of intellect. Why this is so is, at least for the time being, a matter of speculation.

One such speculation offered here is based on the third traditional Chris- tian baseline belief reviewed above, namely, that spirits are more apt to differ in intellect than in will, and that therefore, in its fallen estate–and only in its fallen estate–the body constitutes an even greater impediment to the intellect than to the will. An implication is that the fallen human soul is relatively more capable of willing than of knowing.

This would mean or explain a number of things, such as the following. (a) Humans can love and hate even when they have very little knowledge about the object of their love or hate. (b) Humans are profoundly irrational, because by the very nature of what the term "irrationality" means, it im- plies that the human will is apt to override any amount of knowledge that may be available to it. (c) Humans can come much closer to God via their wills than their intellects. (d) Saying "no" to God, especially if one had received much grace, can become so vehement as to become habitual (Goethe's Lucifer identified himself as "the spirit that always negates"). Such habitual vehemence of the will's negation may generalize to the intellect.

In other words, the soul in its entirety may fall into such a habit of negation, and thus negativism, that the intellect becomes less and less capable of utilizing the potential it has even within the body's limitations. Indeed the body itself may suffer so much from the soul's habitual negation as to devel- op malaise and/or new impediments to the intellect.

For instance, in an effort to shut out God, the body may shut out sensa- tions, perceptions, and the formation of (at least valid) cognitions and infer- ences. A person might literally become (at least "functionally") deaf, blind, etc., and may repress that which does enter the mind into the mind's unconscious. In turn, this alone could render a person "stupid" (in the culturally normative vernacular sense), but that is not even all: it is well known that the process of repression itself consumes vast amounts of psychic energies and that, as a result, repressive personalities exhibit extensive depression of their intellectual efficiency, especially in the areas of attention, concentration, short-term memory, and certain psycho-motor functions.

By the way, conventional professional wisdom may very well be confounded when it has to deal with a person whose "retardation" is the result (or manifestation) of a profound willful resistance to God.

10. Am I then saying that someone can become retarded willfully? Perhaps astonishingly, I would surmise yes, but request that my carefully qualified answer be precisely interpreted. I suspect that someone can willfully become retarded only (a) after first having attained "recognition" of God (i.e., the soul's intellect has glimpsed God), (b) then having directed the will away from God, and then (c) having done at least one of three additional things: having brought about damage to the body so as to delimit further intellectual input to the soul; having brought the will to bear so as to restrict mental input by mentally blocking perceptual pathways; or having repressed relevant psychic content, mostly of a cognitive nature.

I have known persons who seemed to have functioned in the latter mode, i.e., they were mildly or moderately retarded by the usual criteria, had so little consciousness as to seem to be almost sleepwalking, yet showed startling flashes of intellectual capacity–but usually only when wreaking wickedness. Obviously, if such "functional" retardation had its onset still during the childhood of a person, and endured for more than a short period, it might so severely interfere with normal mental growth processes as to become largely irreversible.

11. The above points, and especially so numbers 9 and 10, help one to understand the reality that in most instances, spiritual healing is a precondition to bodily healing, and why people healed of aversion to God may become "smarter."

12. As noted, it has generally been believed that spirits express their existence through their faculties of intellect and will; of course, the soul additionally expresses itself by giving (human) life to a (human) body. While Christ has mysteriously chosen to identify himself deeply with the wounded and rejected people of the world, there is no reason to expect that there should be any relationship (positive or negative) between the "amount" of grace and the amount of natural talent. More likely is that (a) retarded as well as non-retarded people do have callings and missions in life, and (b) retarded people are offered graces, spiritual gifts and charisms commensurate with their callings and missions.

Examples of such callings might be to prophesy, to gentle others, to unite, challenge, confound, convict, etc. (For an elaboration on some of these points, see Wolfensberger, 1977, 1978.) Further, God may act upon others through a retarded person without using the retarded person's intellect or will, but the person's identity, presence, or even movements. To exemplify: God might act upon a person through the gesture–or even mere presence–of another individual whose intellect and will are both so impeded that this individual would be called profoundly retarded.

Potential Misunderstandings

The more a domain is value-laden and emotion-charged, the more likely it is that any phenomenon within, or statement about, this domain will be misunderstood or misinterpreted. Below, I will try (even bend over backwards) to (a) clarify some of my earlier points, and (b) dissociate myself from a series of ideas or interpretations which might conceivably be read into, or derived from, the ideas presented above, especially the proposition that intellectual impairment is much more apt to be associated with volitional impairment than vice versa.

1. People in our era have been so thoroughly misled to think in fallen materialistic quantitative terms that it may bear underlining that merely because a soul's functioning is impeded by its body does not mean that there is "less" of a soul present, or that a person with an impeded soul is any less loved by God.

2. Some retarded people can have strong wills–with all that this implies. However, inflexibility, rigidity, irrational adherence to a stance, stubbornness, etc., though probabilistically (i.e., across populations) related to volition may also derive from other sources (purely material appetitive dynamics, conditioning, etc.), and must not be assumed automatically to be manifestations of the absence of volitional impairment.

3. The above analysis does not mean to imply that all people who end up being considered retarded are incapable of forming meaningful attachments, or of being loving, loyal or unselfish. However, probabilistically, retarded people must be expected to be less capable than non-retarded people of volitional investments of a higher order that rise above the level of our bodily (animal) appetites.

4. Obversely, the above also is not meant to imply that bright people might not have serious volitional deficits. However, it they do have such volitional deficits, these are apt to have at least one additional, and probably much more common, cause: in a non-retarded person, we must expect that much more "schooling" (i.e., training) of the will is possible than in retarded ones, but that lack of such schooling can reduce a non-retarded person to a level of volitional impairment that for practical purposes is no different than that of

many retarded people whose volitional impairment is not due to lack of schooling but to the imperfections of the body.

5. The will may have the capacity to make a fundamental turn toward, or away from God even in some instances where intellect is very severely hampered, and where the person fails to exhibit other signs of a strong will. This helps us to understand the deep spirituality of some very severely retarded persons–and also the perverse obstinacy, defiance, and even outright evil orientation of some similarly impaired people. Benevolently but incorrectly, some observers are inclined to attribute such genuine negative volitional movements of the soul to impairment of the intellect.

However, the fact that even severely retarded people may be capable of fundamental movements of the will is not to imply that everybody is capable of such a fundamental choice toward or away from God. Much as infants may die before attaining a stage (traditionally called the "age of reason") where they can know and choose right from wrong, so a child whose body impedes the intellect may never be able to attain sufficient cognition of God to make a choice, or may die before such cognition has sufficiently developed.

Much controversy has prevailed in Christianity about what happens in such cases, especially if the person is not baptized; the answers have ranged from damnation to limbo to salvation. Considering the eminence of the proponents of all three major positions, I speculatively propose, and with trepidation, that none of them make sense in that they all seem incoherent with "divine style." Limbo, in particular, smacks of a solution more pleasing to the medieval human scholastic intellect than to the "esthetics" of Christian discernment.

Rather, I propose that when a human soul departs the body without having had the opportunity to exercise intellect and will to decide for or against God, God will do what He apparently did with the other spirits, viz., the angels: upon departure from the fallen body and its shackles, God offers the now unimpeded soul a sufficient glimpse of His identity to enable it to make a fundamental choice. It is generally assumed that God offered such a choice to the pure spirits (i.e., angels) upon their creation. Because of the nature of spirits, and because time as we know it is a "temporary" phenomenon expressive of the process of death within (and only within) the fallen domain, the relationship of the angels to God was fixed for eternity the moment their intellects knew and their wills chose. In the extra-fallen domain, there is no "new information" that could sway a spirit's attitude toward God.

Similarly, one might assume that a soul outside the body will immediately have all the "information" "needed" to make an act of the will from which it never retreats because it never even wants to retreat from it. Readers who have taken one of the three "mainline" positions for granted are reminded that some of the most venerable fathers and doctors of the

Church have disagreed with each other on these positions, and that (mostly later) Church councils seemed to have left leeway for the above kind of speculation.

6. Engaging in efforts to fix the fallen universe purely by means of natural, and therefore fallen, means (which I also call "technologies") is commonly but mistakenly perceived, even by truly "good" Christians, as "doing good." A retarded person, especially if also severely physically handicapped, will rarely do much along these lines–which is just as well because such "good" is no good, and merely rearranges the broken pieces of a broken world. The only true good is "fruitful good," which comes from a self-denying submission to Christ which enables a person (or collectivity) to transcend the fall, i.e., to function at least fragmentarily outside the power of Death, and thus possibly also outside the natural laws of the fallen universe.

Such submittal is "being good," but fall-transcending good is rarely acknowledged as good in and by the world; yet such fall-transcending good may indeed be "performed" (actually, mediated) by a retarded person who has sufficient exercise of intellect and will (especially will) to choose God.

7. Although it may appear that the soul of a specific retarded person has been unimpeded enough to make a fundamental movement toward, or away from, God, one is not thereby justified to assume that the person can now be held "responsible" or "accountable" in the usual sense.

In other words, most of us tend to hold to traditional–almost juristic–concepts of responsibility. Unless we are convinced that a person is "insane" (including sufficiently retarded), we are inclined to let the natural consequences of a person's actions take their course, even though these consequences may be disastrous to the person. An extreme example is the new custom in some secular human services of calling the police whenever a retarded client breaks a window, steals something, pulls fire alarms, etc., and to even press charges and prosecute one's retarded clients for minor as well as major infractions. A good number of retarded persons are now in prisons because of this development.

The view presented here is that a retarded person's soul may, in fact, be capable of making a free fundamental choice about its relationship to God, even if that person may be deeply wounded, under great compulsions, or otherwise not really responsible for much of his/her behavior.

Only God can really know what a person is accountable for. Thus, one's assumptions or beliefs about the nature of the choice that has been made by the soul of a retarded person must not become an excuse or justification for one's abandoning, rejecting, or failing to defend or protect that person, or for tolerating or even participating in that person's brutalization. In God's eyes, being kind, serving another person, etc., is meritorious not to the degree that the served person "deserves" it, but to the degree that it contributes to the server's overcoming of the self, to his/her spiritual progress and, thus, to his/her sanctification.

8. None of the above (mostly the discussion of 5 and 7 above) implies an uncritical endorsement of the "holy innocent" interpretation of retarded people. Yes, some retarded people are "innocent" in the sense that they cannot know or choose God or evil at all, or willingly benefit or harm others. Some retarded people are capable of being willfully hurtful and destructive, but they still remain "innocent" in the sense that they act with insufficient knowledge or under much compulsion, and thus will probably not be held accountable by God.

But the idea of "holiness" should probably be reserved for persons (a) whose souls are capable of a free choice, (b) who have chosen God, and (c) who are manifestly endowed with extraordinary graces and gifts. This would include some retarded people, but these would be "innocent" only in a psychological sense, because spiritually, they have known and chosen Good over Evil–which the "innocent" person has not done by virtue of not being able to make a moral choice.

9. None of the above is to endorse either of two mutually opposed mistaken views, namely, (a) that affliction (including retardation) must be assumed to be the result of personal sin (one's own or one's ancestor's), or (b) that it never is. Obviously, one person's (or even nation's) affliction is often the result of an ancestor's (or previous generation's) sins. For instance, a mother's promiscuity or excessive intake of alcohol can cause damage to an unborn child; a nation's warfare can be the cause of the next generation's warfare; etc. Indeed, where retardation was willfully self-inflicted as discussed above, it would be the sinful turning from God that caused such retardation, much as being spiritually healed sometimes results in one's body also being healed.

CONCLUSION

The seven statements presented at the beginning of this article have implications not only to mental retardation, but to other issues at well. For instance, once we understand or believe that the intended state of the human is that of body and soul united in an extra-fallen estate, we can also see more readily that there is a profound illogic in the belief that the soul is infused into the body at any point other than at the moment of the fertilizing union of ovum and sperm.

It is God's will that within the fall (and only within the fall), new human life comes from the tortured, imperfect joining of the issues of man and woman. Once we know that the animal life of humans is not passed on at the moment of coitus but at the moment of fertilization, then a deep comprehension of the reality and nature of the fall (plus possibly other insights) will bring one compellingly to the conclusion that the soul is infused when the life-carrying gametes join to form a cell (i.e., a zygote) that contains within it not only the potential to grow into a mature human, but also to grow into a mature human that is very different from its parent.

Even if a human gamete could be cloned, to do so deliberately seems to do violence to God's design that new human life comes from several levels of a real joining of man and woman, rather than from an ego-centered individual-istic duplication of one's very own animal body–or even an attempt to dupli-cate one's own soul. Indeed, one can even wonder whether human clones are viable; and if so, whether God would grant them human souls.

In the unlikely case that a viable human clone will ever be produced, and if it were a true clone, and if all such clones turned out to lack the capacity to reason abstractly (which seems to also imply that they would lack higher language), then I can see no theological obstacle to the possibility that such a true human clone might be what in the Middle Ages was commonly (and of course mistakenly) called *massa carnis*, i.e., an animal in human shape, much like apes. However, I hasten to dissociate myself from any implication that profoundly retarded (or otherwise handicapped) people (i.e., who are not clones) might (now, in the past, or in the future) lack souls, might therefore not be human, and could therefore be killed without murder being involved. As we know, versions of this view have been advanced as rationales for abortion, infanticide, "euthanasia," genocide, etc.

Some observers (in our time, especially Jean Vanier) have noted that retarded people are creatures of relationship; or relatedly, that love is an especially important language for retarded persons, i.e., persons who are weak in the language and practice of the intellect. In the context of this treatise, these are profoundly relevant observations, though they seem to require some qualification.

What we can probably say along these lines is as follows. (a) Even when a person's capacity to receive communication on the level of the fallen intellect is severely impaired, one can still communicate God's love to that person, and through God's love, also God's word (all this exemplifies fall-transcen-dence). (b) The steadfastness of God's love can be communicated with partic-ular power (i.e., with particularly powerful transcendence of the fall) by a Christian disciple who loves with steadfastness.

In other words, the love of a person who, for and with Christ, enters into a long-term committed love to a retarded person can be expected to com-municate God's love more powerfully to such a retarded person than would the love of the Christian whose love is fragmented, abstract, "prob-abilistic," diffused. Of course, the Spirit is not bound or bindable, and "blows where it listeth" (John 3:8), but the point is that with the occasional exception provided by God for good purpose, retarded people probably have greater need of enduring loving relationships from Christians (yes, "from" more even than "with") than they have need for large numbers of brief loving encounters with numerous Christians. The same need may exist in everybody, but it probably exists to a greater degree in persons of impaired intellect; further, their need may be greater because it is less often met.

We should also note that observations or statements to the effect that retarded people are creatures of relationship does not constitute a contradiction to the earlier assertion that the will of retarded people is often impaired, and their love relationships are often shallower. Indeed, even among non-retarded people, one commonly finds that the weak-willed are more dependent on relationships than those who are actually more capable of forming deeper and more enduring relationships; one might call the former the Marilyn Monroe syndrome. Once more, an implication here is that Christians need to extend steadfast love to retarded people even if that love is not reciprocated, or even if it meets with an inconsistency of response that one may find incomprehensible.

The above considerations are also useful in rejecting some, and supporting and even guiding certain other, developmental and pastoral efforts. At least three ideas are to be rejected.

1. As holy and/or innocent, a (retarded) person who can be presumed to be irrevocably saved has no urgent need of training, bodily amelioration, etc. This belief is wrong because God is life and health, and the closer our union of body and soul comes to its intended full, coherent and healthy functionality, the better. When Jesus healed, He healed body and soul, and improved their unitariness; He did not make people become retarded innocents so that they would be saved for sure.

2. Relatedly, it is wrong to propose that a (retarded) person should be kept from psychological development because mental growth would be apt to enlarge the person's capacity to sin and render him/her susceptible to evil influences and temptations. In reply, the same answer applies as to the enhancement of human life in general. Greater actualization takes place in a universe in which souls are brought to a (greater) capacity to know and choose God, even if some such souls then reject God.

3. Similarly, it is wrong to propose that a retarded person should be kept from contact with the wider world because that world would merely inflict (temporal) harm upon the person. Yes, virtually by definition, a societally devalued person is highly apt to experience devaluing, wrong and hurtful responses in and from the world–but it is also in the context of the larger world that most people carry out their mission in life. Never should anyone

equate the abandoning of a vulnerable person in and to the world with efforts to engage that person deeply and extensively in the life and struggles of society. The retarded person is needed by society as a prophetic sign (Wolfensberger, 1977, 1978, 1979), and efforts to withhold retarded persons from society only in order to spare them potential or actual suffering are illusory (humans cannot guarantee anyone escape from the suffering of a fallen existence), misleading, and injurious to humanity as a whole. However, as needed, the retarded person should be supported, protected, or accompanied by Christian advocates.

Relevant both to Number 2 and 3 above is that a person who is engaged with creation at his/her highest level of capacity has lived more fully even if that life was more suffering. "Abundant life" (John 10:10) surely did not mean a less suffering life!

On the other hand, the above considerations would support approaches which, in addition to well-established pastoral strategies, would attempt to remove bodily impediments (these especially via physical means) to the exercise of intellect and will. Further, of great importance would be the amelioration of sensory functioning in early childhood, the promotion of the development of the child's intellect (which in this case would be much more important than "educating" the child in academic subjects), and the schooling of the child's will. Especially in the case of the latter two strategies, it would be important that they be implemented by people who can also habitually transmit God's love to the child.

These strategies are not new. Many parents, educators of the retarded, and religious shepherds have practiced them, and do so today. Surprisingly, Seguin's own strategy of moral treatment, which he misnamed the "physiological method," was very much along these lines and was related to his own religious faith as a follower of Saint-Simon (1760-1825).[1] However, while many people are "instinctively" doing the right thing, we also see many well-intentioned people acting a bit incoherently in regard to these issues, or even embracing one of the above three errors in toto or in part.

Perhaps the most common error committed by such persons is to depreciate the importance of sharpening a child's intellect and will even while transmitting God's love. Thus, the above consideration might assist such persons in achieving greater validity and coherency in their stance and service.

NOTE

1. Saint-Simon had initially supported a virtual elevation of science to religious status, but changed his mind and identified religion as a prime mover of mankind.

REFERENCES

Wolfensberger, W. The moral challenge of mentally retarded persons to human services. *Information Services* (Publication of the Religion Division of the American Association on Mental Deficiency), 1977, *6* (3) 6-16.

Wolfensberger, W. The prophetic voice and presence of mentally retarded people in the world today. In International Federation of l'Arche (Eds.), *Springs of new hope*. Richmond Hill, Ontario: Daybreak, 1978, 37-80.

Wolfensberger, W. An attempt toward a theology of social integration of devalued/handicapped people. *Information Services* (Publication of the Religion Division of the American Association on Mental Deficiency), 1979, *8*(I), 1226.

How We Carry the Ministry
with Handicapped Persons
to the Parish Level

Wolf Wolfensberger, PhD

In recent years, I have learned that it is impossible to relate validly and coherently to any important aspect of Christianity unless one has a fairly clear understanding of the relationship between creation, fall, redemption, and restoration. It is impossible to understand Christianity unless one understands redemption, and impossible to understand redemption unless one understands the fall. The essence of what I have to say about human services, the place of handicapped people in the world, and ministry by, with, and to handicapped people will be unintelligible unless it is put into this broader context. Yet it is precisely these core truths about creation, fall, redemption, and restoration that are poorly taught in our church today, and in most others. Even worse, one of the reasons these truths are poorly taught is because they are increasingly being rejected, and replaced by what I call "materialized Christianity" that essentially reflects and embraces the false hopes and aspirations of our materialistic culture rather than the true–and indeed only–hopes that God offers.

Because of these realities, I will briefly sketch an orthodox but currently minority Christian view of history:

The crucial historical timelines for a Christian: (A) Creation, (B) Fall,

Reprinted with permission from *National Apostolate with Mentally Retarded Persons Quarterly*, 1983, 14, 9, 12-13, (summary of a presentation at the 13th annual conference of the National Apostolate with Mentally Retarded Persons, Denver, 10 August 1983). Presentation condensed by Father Charles L. Hughes.

[Haworth co-indexing entry note]: "How We Carry the Ministry with Handicapped Persons to the Parish Level." Wolfensberger, Wolf. Co-published simultaneously in *Journal of Religion, Disability & Health* (The Haworth Pastoral Press, an imprint of The Haworth Press, Inc.) Vol. 4, No. 2/3, 2001, pp. 85-90; and: *The Theological Voice of Wolf Wolfensberger* (ed: William C. Gaventa, and David L. Coulter) The Haworth Pastoral Press, an imprint of The Haworth Press, Inc., 2001, pp. 85-90.

(C) Redemption, (D) Restoration. The fall resulted in an alienation from God of everything human, plus everything over which humans were meant to exercise dominion, and a secondary rupture of all relationships within creation. All this is especially apparent in four manifestations: (1) The corruption and distortion of the identities of creatures, (2) Dislocation of the place (locale) of creatures into fallen space, (3) Distortion and disruption of relationships among creatures, (4) Dislocation of creation into fallen time.

A major overarching consequence of the fall is that nothing that is done on the fallen level, and by humans using only their own fallen human identities and powers, "works right." Christians, including our own theological authorities, are commonly deluded in that they see the fall manifested primarily in individual human sinfulness, pride, lust, vice, greed, etc. They commonly fail to recognize that any collective human enterprise is just as fallen as any individual is–and in some respects even more so because such enterprises are even less under human control than the individual human is. Collective entities and efforts, because of their characteristics such as complexity, unconsciousness, and irrationality, rapidly slip under demonic control. They become principalities and powers, and they become demonically-controlled regardless of the goodness or badness of their members or leaders.

Some of the manifestations of the dysfunctionality of the world:

1. Humans are imperfect, will remain so, and will never control the universe.
2. Humans will always suffer hardships as a result of disturbances and upheavals in the physical world.
3. There will always be social devaluation on both the individual and collective levels.
4. Physical force: (A.) Operates throughout the universe, (B.) Becomes violence when used among people, (C.) Will always be used among people
5. Every good scheme that humans create will eventually become perverted.
6. Because of their complexity, organizations and social institutions will be especially subject to perversion.
7. "Caesar," or the state, will always pretend to be, or try to be, God.

In essence, many of these dysfunctionalities reflect ongoing human idolatry, and misplaced trust and hope.

Redemption is the first of two steps God has mysteriously and graciously chosen for His restoration of all human-related creation to its originally intended state: Redemption is not restoration, but the granting to the followers of Christ of (a) partial, and (b) temporally limited, fragments of those powers which humans had prior to the fall, and which the redeemed will possess fully after their restoration. These powers enable Christians to "transcend the fall," i.e., be or do things which are above or outside the fall. These powers include the charismata, i.e., the gifts of the Spirit, which are no less than fragments of our true–as distinguished from our "natural"–human identities, powers and vocation in what I call the "extra-fallen" state. While these "empowerments" (as I also call them) are granted to individual believers, they are especially generously granted to Christian communalities. However, since fallen humans do not possess these powers naturally, they are expressions of the divine, i.e., of the Holy Spirit, working in and through the Christian. These powers are granted only to Christians, and largely in proportion to how much they have given up their idols, acknowledged their own powerlessness, ergo "denied their very selves" (Matthew 16:24; Mark 8:34; Luke 9:23), and permitted God to work through them in their own stead. It is God who takes over when we function above the fall, usually either by giving us infused knowledge or power that is of the image of God, and that permits us to emit an act representative of our true extra-fallen identity. This is what Christ has enabled his followers to do through his redemption, and what He calls them to do.

One of the implications of the redemptive act is that Christians, i.e., those who accept the offered redemption, are invited to live now, still within the midst of the fall, and even still under the power of Death, as if the restoration had already taken place. God has promised that those who do this in faith will be sustained in doing it.

Obviously, trying to live now as if one lived outside the fall does not mean that one is as yet fully restored, but one will receive sufficient grace to at least fragmentally transcend the fall, and one will be sufficiently fruitful to be a witness to seeking souls (including other Christians), and a scandal to those who are adamantly opposed to God (including some professed Christians).

This has a number of implications which we can identify. They all derive from an analysis of what life in paradise is apt to be like.

1. Restored people follow their vocation. They strive to do what God created them to be and do.
2. The main thing people were created to do, and therefore the main thing that people in paradise do, is delight so much in their vision of and communion with God that they praise Him continually. Accordingly, we here on earth should strive toward a similar state of mind, being, and acting.

While not everybody in paradise would be identical or even "equal," as we understand the term, everybody there would be in perfect harmony with everyone else. In turn, this would mean or imply the following:

1. The unity of the Body of Christ should, on earth, mirror the paradisial perfection of that unity. Thus, Christians should seek equivalent harmony among each other now.

2. The paradisial harmony is among the saints, but not between them and the demons or lost souls. Similarly, harmony among the followers of Christ on earth does not mean that there should not or will not be conflict with demonic principalities and powers, or even with people not yet submitted to Christ.

The foregoing thinking helps us to see more clearly what the unity of the Body of Christ is all about.

Some realities or implications of the unity of the Body of Christ:

1. The importance of Christian communality is one of the most central aspects of Christianity.
2. It is most difficult to lead a Christian life outside a primary Christian community.
3. Special powers adhere to acting within the Christian communality, and in a Christian collective context.
4. Members of a Christian communality support each other at least as much as an old-fashioned extended family used to.
5. Members' commitment to, and support of, each other surpasses that extended to other groups to which they belong.
6. Each member of the body is seen as contributing to it in some way.
7. Members' spiritual gifts and natural talents should be nourished and capitalized upon.
8. A member can legitimately lay all sorts of claims on the body.
9. The communality will go to great lengths to avoid the expulsion of a member.
10. Member exclusion is damaging to the rest of the body especially if it damages the member who is excluded.

Several of the above points imply that Christians should not engage in either imposed or self-selected divisions of their communal bodies along irrelevant lines. Relevant are mostly such things as the validity of one's faith, the gifts of the Spirit, including the various gifts of ministry, and harmony within the body. Irrelevant are most of people's personal characteristics, including their handicaps. Similarly, Christians should not segregate their members on the basis of irrelevant characteristics. Where some sort of segregation seems absolutely necessary, it should be kept to the minimum. However, that which is necessary should not be determined on the basis of a fallen calculus (e.g., how likely it is to "work," how costly or inexpensive it is, how productive/contributive a person is, how demanding a person is), but on the basis of communal submission in faith and trust in God.

What we have covered so far has implications in turn, such as the following:

Some implications of the unity of the body of Christ to participation and formation on the level of the congregation or Christian community:

1. The community puts its faith in Christian transcendence of the fall, rather than in fallen technologies.
2. The Christian communality considers it normative to stand in contradiction to the practices of the world (e.g., in regard to inclusion of people who are devalued/at risk), and characteristics/behaviors of members that elicit segregation in the world do not do so in the Christian body, where extraordinary efforts are made to enable maximally feasible inclusion and participation of members at risk.
3. The community bends over backward to establish positive roles for members at risk of devaluation/rejection.
4. The community defends a member at risk from afflictions and external oppression.
5. Generally every effort is made to serve the needs of a member within the basic community before the person is sent to another Christian service.
6. If a vulnerable person can only receive a non-Christian service technology by being severed from a Christian community, then the technical benefits should be foregone.
7. Where a degree of segregation within/from the basic community seems unavoidable, every effort is made to keep it to the minimum.
8. Address of non-member or far-off needs before urgent needs of members are addressed symptomatizes a failure of the basic Christian communality.
9. Christian formation must follow, not precede, valued communal participation of members.

While all human services rendered on the fallen level are technologies that can yield no fruit, the services which Christians render in a fall-transcending fashion become ministries, i.e., service and ministry that are fall-transcendingly unified and can bear fruit. However, we need to be clear that Christian human service is God working through the "spiritual transparency" of the server. Thus, the service must primarily be service to oneself, in the sense that it is part of one's struggle to follow Jesus to holiness. Ordinarily, no fruit can come of any act that is not sanctifying to the actor.

As service is transformed into ministry, it brings both body and soul of the server closer to their divinely-intended harmony with each other and with God, and the very same fruit is offered to the person served if she/he will only be open to the Spirit of God. It is by means of mutual ministry that we transact a major portion of Christian communality. Those who do little or no ministry are at best on the margins of a Christian communality. This applies fully to handicapped or otherwise afflicted people. Afflictions are in the fallen domain, but charismata are not. Ergo, handicapped people can be expected to have their full share of the gifts of the Holy Spirit, and afflicted and handicapped Christians whose souls are turned to God can be expected to be able to minister to others the same as, though perhaps in different ways than, other Christians can.

We can spell out some increasingly specific implications. Assuming that a local congregation proceeds properly–and very few do–then we can further assume that eventually it will be able to serve all its members in such a fashion that none need to be separated from the communality, or to enter into major or chronic dependency on non-Christian service entities. In time, the local congregation can develop the following pattern of service ministry components.

Some service modalities by which a local church can serve its own members:

1. Eliciting part-time or voluntary service from members and others, and providing a mechanism for matching volunteers, tasks and people in need.
2. People sharing homes with each other: (a) Opening one's own home to needy person(s), (b) Living supportively in the home of needy person(s), (c) Creating a mutual joint home.
3. Members finding work, training and employment positions for other members, or mediating such.
4. Recruitment of full-time workers ("Deacons") at little or no pay, probably implying at least temporary voluntary poverty.
5. Appeal for life-time service (as "Deacons"), usually implying voluntary poverty.
6. A discreet informal diaconal almonership.
7. If unavoidable, operate certain "services": (a) Work projects for training and/or (subsidized) employment, with special emphasis on neighborhood improvement, (b) Hostels, hospices and houses of healing if within the congregation's boundaries, and by/for the members, (c) Other services, e.g., Christian counseling.

The Most Urgent Issues Facing Us as Christians Concerned with Handicapped Persons Today

Wolf Wolfensberger, PhD

On his wandering through Palestine, Jesus endlessly performed miracles. Yet some Pharisees and Sadducees came to Him and asked for a miracle, to prove His authenticity. Jesus answered, "When the sun is setting you say 'It is going to rain, because the sky is red and dark.' You can predict the weather by looking at the sky; but you cannot interpret the signs concerning these times!" (Mt. 16:1-4).

The faithful Christian pilgrim tries to hear God's call. I propose that the biggest single question such pilgrims must ask today is: what time do we live in, and what does this time call for? What one believes about the answer to this question determines the stance one takes vis-à-vis all important issues of the day, including strategies related to service issues in regard to mentally retarded persons.

One's reading of the signs of the times can be facilitated by several reflections:

1. Not every phenomenon is a sign of its times.
2. Some phenomena are signs of universal realities and truths rather than of their specific times.
3. Signs of the times are usually clusters of phenomena that are quintessentially and simultaneously (a) defining of a major important moral reality and (b) portents of important realities to come. Often they an-

Reprinted with permission from an abbreviation of a presentation at the 13th annual conference of the National Apostolate with Mentally Retarded Persons, Denver, 10 August 1983; published in *National Apostolate with Mentally Retarded Persons Quarterly*, 1983, *14*(3), 4-9. Condensed by Dr. Robert R. Lebel.

[Haworth co-indexing entry note]: "The Most Urgent Issues Facing Us as Christians Concerned with Handicapped Persons Today." Wolfensberger, Wolf. Co-published simultaneously in *Journal of Religion, Disability & Health* (The Haworth Pastoral Press, an imprint of The Haworth Press, Inc.) Vol. 4, No. 2/3, 2001, pp. 91-102; and: *The Theological Voice of Wolf Wolfensberger* (ed: William C. Gaventa, and David L. Coulter) The Haworth Pastoral Press, an imprint of The Haworth Press, Inc., 2001, pp. 91-102.

nounce an ending, and usually also a beginning (or at least an increase) of something else.

4. Signs can be directed at all of humankind, or at particular sectors (nations, classes, etc.).
5. Most signs are unusual at least in the sense that they would have been viewed as unusual at an earlier time.
6. Whether a sign is good or bad does not determine the goodness or badness of that to which it points. Scripture has told us that almost all the signs pointing to the fervently desired second coming of Jesus will be unpleasant.
7. Signs of the times more often point to bad than to good developments, and specifically to patterns of human immorality and rebellion against God. This should not be the least bit surprising, since we live in fallen time.
8. Since the signs commonly point to human sinfulness, they can also be understood as calls to repentance.
9. The biggest obstacle to reading the signs of the times is idolatry, i.e., having excessive attachments to things created rather than to the Creator.
10. Conversely, the more one is able to detach from the world because one is secure in the trust of God, the more apt one is to read the signs and perceive their meaning.

At almost any time, important truths are unpopular, often because they are unpleasant and discomforting, especially to the established powers. We are carefully taught not to read the signs of our times. Those who tell time are rejected, even martyred (Mt 5:11-12; Lk 6:23; 11:47-48; 13:34; Acts 7:52; Rom 11:8).

Following are some seventeen signs of our times as I perceive them:

1. This age has achieved unprecedented understanding of the intricacies of the universe, and unprecedented technological capabilities. This includes dramatic breakthroughs in three crucial areas: (a) biology and especially molecular genetics, (b) cosmology, aided by space travel, and (c) nuclear physics. Unfortunately, all of this is being accomplished with unbridled Promethean arrogance. The intellectual classes are laying a claim to God-like mastery over creation, acknowledging no restraint over their work, and evidencing no respect for moral authority greater than theirs. This is idolatry.

2. It is the technology just mentioned that is bringing about a dramatic change-over in the modes of production, distribution and consumption of goods and services. The more "developed" a nation becomes, the more this means that it is using less and less of its manpower for, first, agricultural production, and secondly other primary production such as manufacture and construction. In turn, this means that the age-old pyramid of labor is increasingly turned upside down.

3. The very technology that liberates people from toil with soil, nature,

animals and tools has also resulted in alienations from hand labor and the recognition that ultimately all wealth derives from labor.

4. Closely connected to this is an alienation from nature. Multigenerational urbanization divests people of contact with nature, the experience of weather being long-distance and sheltered.

5. Europe, and all westernized societies that derive therefrom, were founded on Judeo-Christian traditions, principles, values and religious forms that became incorporated into the Roman empire after 325 A.D. On three continents, these principles have been at least idealized and aspired to, albeit ineffectually. Yet in a single generation we have seen the repudiation of 1700 years of this fabric of civilization, and most importantly of its ideals. This includes the traditional connections between morality and law, deterioration of which is apparent in the rapid changes in law and legal practice pertaining to sexuality, marriage, family, parent-child relations, the nature of human-hood, abortion, and euthanasia of the ill and afflicted.

6. That which symbolizes this repudiation should not be confused with that which replaces it. For example, the fascination with eastern cults and gurus is mostly just a symptom of repudiation of the Judeo-Christian tradition. More, it is a replacement with a value cluster which, regardless of what name or guise it may be given, is a very logically intertwined materialistic, individualistic, hedonistic utilitarianism. This involves several components and results: (a) a turning away from the world of the spirit and from metaphysical belief systems, (b) an increased preoccupation with the material, (c) rejection of a metaphysics typically resulting in a very logical idolization of the human and exaltation of the individual; (d) idolization of human intellect and its products; (e) religious belief in a mythical entity called "progress"; (f) unbridled individualism and selfishness; construction of ethical values on the basis of utilitarianism . . . . "situation ethics"; (g) an attitude of entitlement to whatever one wants; (h) a belief of quasi-religious proportions that afflictions, suffering and even minor hardships are evil and that they must and will be eliminated; (i) a belief that one is entitled to freedom from affliction and suffering; (j) a surrender to what one can call hedonism, i.e., exaggerated and uninhibited aspirations to comfort.

7. Out of the technological developments mentioned above has arisen an unprecedented capacity for mankind to inflict death in the world, and that in multiple ways. Indeed, just as we claim divine mastery over creation (by intellectual advances in genetics, cosmology and nuclear physics), we find ourselves producing the means of destroying life (including ourselves) on a global scale. This is a supreme irony. We are facing significant dangers from the proliferation of nuclear weapons, the contamination of our environment by nuclear wastes, the application of genetic engineering techniques, the

development of germ and chemical weaponry, advances toward climate control, and the multiplicities of pollution.

8. As a corollary to the above trends, I increasingly see phenomena that I call "alliances with death," by which I mean that a collectivity commits its very identity to the wreaking of death in the world, to inflicting it on a large scale over the long run, to using it as a major means toward its other goals, and even to celebrating death in such a fashion as to bring that collectivity's own death about. As one example of what may very well be the beginning of a death alliance: for the first time in almost 3000 years, the medical profession has severed its ties from its traditional and unswerving commitment to the preservation and protection of life, and has permitted itself to become an executioner: foremost in abortion, but also in infanticide, in so-called "euthanasia," and in the medicalization of capital punishment.

9. Societies have always had ways of drastically cutting off their unproductive and/or burdensome members, such as unwanted newborns and the feeble aged. However, Judeo-Christian ideals have always been opposed to such homicidal practices, though it often offered understanding when such practices took place under conditions of dire distress, extreme poverty, famine, migration, etc. But today, despite their Judeo-Christian tradition, the wealthiest nations are among the leaders in the practice of legalizing and performing abortion, infanticide, "euthanasia," and various disguised ways of inflicting death upon their devalued classes. Indeed, we can almost speak of a wave of hatred toward procreation, unborn children, and even children in general and the marriage institution as a potential locus of procreation.

One of my major missions at this time is to reveal the extent to which genocide of handicapped and afflicted people is in progress, and to call for its repudiation. Not counting abortions, I estimate that in the United States alone, the number of afflicted or devalued people who die each year because their lives were taken outright, or whose lives were at least very significantly abbreviated, can easily amount to 200,000. I have publicly and frequently spoken on this issue, yet my well-documented message is almost totally ignored, even by the very class of people that is here today. The relative indifference of the Catholic Church to this phenomenon is comparable to its low opposition to the killing of the Jews and the handicapped people in Europe by the Nazis. These three shameful realities are themselves signs of our times.

10. The trends discussed so far must also be considered in the light of the fact that human progress in the areas of psychology, sociology, and communications has enabled the principalities of the world to accumulate unprecedented powers. This is apparent in multiple domains:

   a. The existence of super-powers, such as the United States and USSR,
   b. The power of the military arms of even relatively minor and small nations, which is such today that they would be able to easily defeat the super-powers of a century ago,

    c. The manipulation of language, imagery and consciousness is so so-
       phisticated as to enable worldly powers to deeply influence or even
       control people's opinions, politics, religion, lifestyle and economic
       behavior,
    d. Means of identification, surveillance and tracking of people have
       become very powerful,
    e. There are now powerful means of chemical mind control, e.g., tran-
       quilizers to keep devalued minorities quiet.

The above means are used by some bodies to control their own members
or to subjugate others, and they may also be used very effectively to "detoxi-
fy" or hide grave evils that are being committed.

    11. One problem that science and technology have brought is unprecedent-
ed complexity. Almost any human, and certainly almost any collective enterprise has grown more complex, commonly to the point where systems can be
viewed as pyramids standing on their tips. Complexity implies many things,
including greater specialization, fewer well-rounded people, failures are
more catastrophic, failures of entire systems result from failure of small
elements of the system, systems are disabled with greater ease, etc. The more
complex things become, the less they are under human control, the more they
fall under demonic control, and the less recognizable are the malfunctions
and evils of the system.

    12. Several of the trends mentioned include elements of oppression, but
yet another new element is the degree of sophistication of oppression which
has increased with the complexity of things, the developments in communications, and the debasement of language. As a result, the ruling strata of the
world today can oppress the poor with such subtlety that the reality of the
oppression escapes the notice of many of the oppressors and oppressed alike.

    All this has enabled evils in the world to not only become more systematic,
but to conceal their identity. For instance, there is relatively little awareness
of four major patterns of oppression in the world. (a) The wealth of the more
developed nations is substantially supported by the (sometimes irreversible)
extraction of resources from the poor ones. (b) Even in developed nations, the
twenty percent or so of the people who are the very producers of the wealth
that the rest enjoy are largely on the economic bottom. The most striking
examples are farmers and peasants. (c) The manufacture of devalued people
in developed countries to employ human service workers. (d) Massive genocide of handicapped people so that hardly anyone will perceive the phenomenon as such, label it as such, or address it as such.

    13. We can point to a number of major stresses on modern society that are
largely the results of a feedback loop set in motion by technologization and
materialization. These stresses all involve momentous and unprecedentedly

rapid changes in the way people live, and in their social institutions. They include the following:

a. A weakening or even collapse of virtually every single bond that can bind people together into a polity. This includes virtually all social institutions, including sex-gender coherency, marriage, family, esteem across generations and sexes, mutual trust, etc. In our society, the law is barely managing to function, and is already as much a disabler as a facilitator of society.

b. Cultural shock, insofar as the pace of change has so quickened that virtually every custom, tradition and belief have come under attack, including those that have prevailed for thousands of years and yet are often overthrown in a fraction of a lifetime. This is exemplified in phenomena such as for the first time in human history, youngsters being apt to know more than their elders, contributing to divisiveness among age groups and family breakdown.

c. An unprecedented and phenomenal increase in population in certain parts of the world.

d. Uprooting and dislocation of people, especially as rural folk fall prey to the lying promises of materialism and move to the cities, there to disintegrate socially, lose millennia of their culture, and often starve or otherwise die.

e. Urbanization and crowding of gargantuan proportions, as exemplified by Mexico City which is predicted to grow to 31 million people.

We should note that the stressful changes that have been occurring involve an extensive weakening of the very conventions and institutions that have been sources of continuity, strength, a sense of belonging, mutual support and security to people.

On the religious scene there have also been momentous discontinuities. Some seem related to the dynamics mentioned above, some may derive from more direct divine intervention.

14. Many parts of the world are witnessing an unprecedented increase in the formalization of societal processes, human relationships, human services, law, etc. This development has multiple roots, including the following: (a) It represents a frantic response of people and institutions to the increasing complexity and unmanageability of things. People imagine that with greater objectification, fractionation, redistribution, prescription, etc., of processes, tasks and roles, complexity can be managed. (b) It is part of the process by which worldly empires try to increase or maintain power and control over affairs.

For example, the Holocaust differed from earlier genocides in history not only in its magnitude, but in the way it was brought about, namely, by mustering the processes of a systematic, scientificated bureaucratism that objectified the killing and broke it down into its components in such a fashion that it was able to elicit the collaboration, or at least the collusion, of literally hundreds of millions of people, including vast numbers of those who would have opposed it had it been carried out in an overt, bloody, passionate way in their midst: In other words, bureaucratization succeeded superbly in making mass violence "clean," "neat" and normative, and in converting it from a bloody, undisciplined, sporadic personal or mob event into an objectified, systematized, disciplined and even unbloody operation which could be manipulated from afar.

Interpreters of the Holocaust also point out that this extermination was "legitimate"–perhaps not in every technical legal aspect, but in its broader aspects. After all, there had been a systematic legalization of discrimination, it was the government that carried out the program, it was its officials (including the courts) that upheld it, it was the medical profession and the people who collaborated or colluded in it, and it was the churches and other moral authorities that generally remained silent against it.

All the above explains why there was so little opposition to both the Holocaust and to the concomitant destruction of handicapped people, and why hardly any of the participants ever repented of their parts.

15. Some of the developments I mentioned are much more apparent in some societies than others, but one striking phenomenon of our day is a convergence of the world to a certain homogeneity, namely to an industrialized technologized materialistic hedonism. Regardless whether the professed ideology is Christianity, Communism, Buddhism, Islam, humanism or whatever, the de facto aspiration of less-developed societies is to become like the developed West. I call this development "mundality," and view it as a very logical and realistic outcome of what is bound to happen in a world that moves toward what Teilhard de Chardin envisioned as planetized collective cerebralization, except that Teilhard envisioned it as an idealized "noosphere" with an Omega Point, whereas in a fallen world, all we can expect is a demonically grinning caricature thereof, for which "mundality" is a much more apt name.

16. Personally, I have concluded that one of the really big signs of our times is profound mass insanity. In a complex feedback loop, it is hard to say what is cause, effect, or correlate. In part, people do some of the things sketched above because they are crazy, but in bigger part I believe that these things have made them crazy. Sensorium is blunted or blocked, intellect derailed, language utterly incoherent and tongues confounded, passions deadened, the will weakened, etc. I see this craziness as not only a personal one but also as pervading entire collectivities, organizations, nations, churches, universities, etc., etc. Indeed, I believe we are witnessing mundality of insanity of gigantic proportions.

17. In a fallen world, Christianity was meant to be a light to the pagans, a model to the confused, and a rock of never-changing truth. Yet I would say that this is a time of possibly unprecedented moral confusion within Christianity and within the Catholic Church. The flock is confused about war and peace, nuclear arms and nuclear power, the nature and role of the sexes, the family and divorce, attitudes toward the environment, toward genetics, toward life and death, toward contraception, abortion, infanticide and euthanasia. The flock is confused in good part because the shepherds are confused. They speak like the scribes, without authority. Perhaps as never before, pronunciations on matters of faith and morals coming from the moral authorities of the Church (priests, monks and nuns, professors of theology and ethics, even bishops) may be no different than those coming from the secular sector, and thus have to be subjected to the same skeptical analysis as the latter.

Now I will attempt to interpret the meaning of these signs of our times.

1. Insofar as these developments have little or no precedent, and considering that there are so many of them, I believe that we live in an extraordinarily unique era.
2. One thing that all these 17 developments seem to have in common is an idolatrous exaltation of the human, and especially of those human attributes that have to do with either intellect, will, or power. Intellect is exalted in the promotion of technology and industry, will in the exaltation of individualism, and power in the development of mechanisms for controlling or destroying people. The human race is recapitulating the fall and building yet another tower of babel, and yet once again, the Lord is confounding minds and tongues.
3. Many of these signs herald not only a possibly uniquely rapid collapse of a major culture, but especially a cataclysmic collapse of Judeo-Christian tradition, at least of the Occidental type.
4. The signs overwhelmingly point toward nuclear war.
5. The signs also are powerfully suggestive that we are living at the end of times. The end, as it is sometimes called, is actually merely the end of fallen time, and the reinstitution of the intended divine order. As such, it is to be eagerly anticipated rather than dreaded. The only thing to dread is the remainder of fallen time. Without promoting concretistic interpretations of apocalyptic scripture, I find some passages highly applicable (Matthew 24:5, 10-13, and 28:19; Luke 24:47 and 21:27).

Personally, I believe that the Parousia is more imminent than at any other time since the Redemption. If it is imminent, and if "only" nuclear war were, we should expect extraordinary prophetic manifestations, most likely including not only the rise of individual prophets, but also of entire prophetic Christian communities or movements, and possibly other signs. Alert Christians would be actively looking for these signs so as to benefit therefrom. While no one knows the day or the hour, we were told that signs of Christ's return would be given, and that these signs were readable, though of course they would not necessarily be widely read.

One possible prophetic sign in my opinion has been the assumption of a prophetic identity by so many retarded people in our time. I have elaborated on this in a lengthy paper elsewhere ("The Moral Challenge of Mentally Retarded Persons to Human Services," *Information Services*, Newsletter of Religion Division, American Association on Mental Deficiency (1977) 6 (3): 6-16; and *Springs of Hope,* Daybreak Publications, Richmond Hill, Ontario, Canada, International Federation of L'Arche (1978) p. 37-80). I propose that the abundant prophetic presence and behavior of retarded people in society today is (a) evidence of God's derision of the current human intellectual arrogance as manifested especially in science and technology, and (b) a harbinger of God's impending termination of that arrogance.

I also perceive a possible sign in the recent, and sometimes dramatic, drawing together of devout Christians of diverse denominations on the local level, and/or in joint undertakings. I am not speaking of what is happening on the level of the administration of denominations, or official joint study commissions, or merger talks, but of small, intimate, genuine joining in genuine Christian tasks. I interpret this development not so much as a harbinger of official mergers of denominations, but as a divine preparation of the faithful few for days of tribulation ahead when the faithful will no longer be able to communicate with their higher church centers and authorities far away, but will instead draw together with each other in the face of adversity, and where the common bond of submission to the Holy Spirit will be stronger than the differences in denominational identities.

The children of this age have been so corrupted by modernism that they want only "good news," and because they want good news only on their own materialistic terms, they fail to hear any genuinely good news that they are given. Their thinking has also often been so taken over by modern materialistic paradigms of quantitative thought that if they are given ten messages of bad news and five of good, they are left under the impression that bad news is "winning," and/or that the good news is somehow insufficient. Thus, I can clearly hear the plaintive and even accusatory query in response to the above exposition, "But have you no good news? Is everything bad? Is there no hope?"

There is indeed little hope if people who have been given good news ask for good news. However, for those who may have had difficulty separating the good from the bad news I will extract the major points of good news.

1. The old imperial arrangements of the world are coming to an end.
2. We are seeing more starkly how bankrupt and empty are the hopes of the world, and therefore can rejoice even more in the true hopes to which we as Christians are called.

3. God is confounding the minds, thoughts and language of the proud and mighty who wanted to build a tower to heaven and take it over.
4. The Lord is sending us prophets, prophecy and saints specifically for our age.
5. God is exalting many of the littlest people of the earth, such as the native peasants in poverty-stricken areas that are forming charismatic base communities and proclaiming God's truth to the mighty; mentally retarded people who are serving as prophets to an intellectually bankrupt world.
6. On a personal level, devout Christians are overcoming their denominational divisions, and drawing closer together.
7. Christ's second coming, the deliverance of the faithful, and the restoration of all things to their pre-fallen harmony may be close at hand.

I have always believed that proper formulation of an issue will commonly imply what action is indicated. Many Christian responses to some of the signs of the times seem to me to be obvious. However, I will highlight several:

1. Those who desire to be Christians need to orient themselves vigorously vis-à-vis (a) time, and (b) place. In other words, they need to start telling time, ergo reading the clocks; and they need to plant their feet on firm ground, consisting not only of orthodox Christian faith and morals, but also of their gifts of the Spirit, their mission in life, and their primary Christian communal bodies.

2. To help us orient ourselves, we need to identify what and who can help us. This includes orienting ourselves to who the prophets are of our day, what the prophetic movements are and what their significance is, and which Christian communalities are functioning charismatically, i.e., under the genuine guidance of the Holy Spirit, rather than under the fallen laws of human groups and formal organizations.

Also, in the sea of confusion, babel, rebellion against God and discontinuity, it is essential to have one of one's anchors in a committed Christian communality. Since many of you are in Holy Orders, I hasten to add that this is not necessarily enough, since even persons in Holy Orders may not function communally, and some religious communities no longer function even Christianly.

3. A valid internal orientation will usually imply an externally visible mission. The hardship of such missions is apt to parallel the hardship of the times.

The members of this organization specifically need to ask themselves whether they believe that these are cataclysmic times, and if so, whether cataclysmic times do not call for patterns of response that differ from those that one might emit at other times–even other troublesome times. If one agrees that these are cataclysmic times, then one should ask whether and how the things one is doing differ from those one would otherwise have done. How members view the times can be strongly inferred by scanning the organization's publications.

4. We must say a vigorous "no" to the non-Christian assumptions and values of the world, and a "no" to its attempts to control our language and minds. We must be most skeptical vis-à-vis the modern idioms of communication, and confront them with "kingdom idiom." This has special implications in the context of human service and societally devalued people, because concepts and language there have become so thoroughly corrupted.

Again, one of the implications specifically to this organization and its members is that they need to be much more critical of the dominant realities and structures, the schemes these structures spawn, the style they adopt, etc. This organization should play much more the role of a critic and dismantler of the prevailing order than one that endorses or even apes it. Indeed, one needs to examine not only whether "the world" requires critique and dismantling, but whether elements of church life do as well.

5. Because we live under the shadow of global death, we all need to confront and combat the Satanic feast. We must do that in at least four ways.

   a. We must develop a coherent stance on life as a whole, and become competent in understanding and explaining the relevant issues and dynamics.

   b. In a world that is rushing headlong into unimaginable mass destruction, it is high time–maybe even last chance–for the church to return to its early, and to the only valid, commitment to life, and to repudiate, triumphantly as well as penitentially, its own 1500 years of alliance with violence and death. We need to acknowledge that Christ called us to be non-violent, and try to convert this acknowledgment into our lives and politics, including our stances toward all forms of deathmaking.

God is a God of life. It is only through Satan that death is transacted into the world. Life is unitary, death is unitary and the two forces are opposed to each other. One of the things this means is that we need to see the underlying unity and continuity of actions that promote death in the world. Because our consciences and consciousness have been so blinded, we do not even have a relevant language for some of these realities, which is why I use the term "deathmaking" to refer to such a broad range of phenomena.

   c. We need to take a stand against the genocides of our time, and especially that of the unborn and handicapped that has broken out in our time. The more a group of people come under oppression, the more important is it that Christians come to their aid, and stand in solidarity with them. This holds true especially for any Christian who has a special relationship, calling, or mission in relation to such an oppressed group. Thus, for us here, this would mean a vigorous engagement on the issue, proclaiming the truth to others, and defending those at risk. This means actions both on behalf of specific individuals at risk, as well as on the level of principle and collectivity.

In the small space I have, I could not begin to document and explain the genocidal warfare that has broken out against many classes of societally devalued people in our society, and in much of the West. This is one of the most urgent issues for people such as ourselves. We need to become highly informed of the realities, understand their origins and dynamics, and be able to address the developments in a Christian fashion, with the vigor and vehemence they deserve. Today, it is not good enough to even be convinced of the issue; it is also necessary to be competent in understanding its dynamics.

d. We must cultivate our love of creation, even though it is fallen. This includes a preservation of species and resources, and other practices of good stewardship over the world and its creatures.

6. It is time for Christians to detach themselves from the imperial human service super-system, to confront it, to pronounce judgment over it, and to construct Christian alternatives. These alternatives consist primarily of three major strategies: informal personal friendship and advocacy relationships between impaired and other people, informal Christian communalities of such people, and formation of radical Christian local congregations where the needs of members are met by or through fellow members. These latter two should be assimilative of afflicted people, by which I do not mean that they are communities of or for handicapped people, but of Christians in general who will assimilate a proportion of handicapped persons as members. Regarding retarded persons specifically, they even more than other people need an atmosphere of kindness and spiritual nurture in order to unfold their spirituality and practice their charismatic gifts.

The Good Life
for Mentally Retarded Persons

Wolf Wolfensberger, PhD

I was once asked to define what might be "the good life" for mentally retarded persons. The concept of the "good life" goes back at least to the classical period of Greek philosophy, and was controverted by greats such as Plato. The question is clearly a challenging one, and as important as it is, people who carry a major responsibility in, or even for, the lives of mentally retarded individuals rarely explicate in a conscious and coherent fashion their vision of the good life for such persons. From the perspective of the prevailing materialistic world view, the good life for retarded persons would probably have to be defined entirely in terms of material and emotional welfare. However, I will attempt to delineate the issue from a Christian perspective; within such a perspective, considerations of material and emotional welfare are important issues, but not ultimate ones.

BASELINE ASSUMPTIONS

I begin with one major baseline assumption, namely, that there is no reason to expect that the criteria for the good life of mentally retarded persons should be drastically different from those for people in general. Once one accepts this assumption, then it becomes all the more surprising that when confronted with the challenge of defining the good life for retarded persons, people are apt to stutter a bit and perhaps give incoherent or incomplete answers.

Reprinted with permission from *National Apostolate with Mentally Retarded Persons Quarterly* Publication, 1984, *15*(3), 18-20.

[Haworth co-indexing entry note]: "The Good Life for Mentally Retarded Persons." Wolfensberger, Wolf. Co-published simultaneously in *Journal of Religion, Disability & Health* (The Haworth Pastoral Press, an imprint of The Haworth Press, Inc.) Vol. 4, No. 2/3, 2001, pp. 103-109; and: *The Theological Voice of Wolf Wolfensberger* (ed: William C. Gaventa, and David L. Coulter) The Haworth Pastoral Press, an imprint of The Haworth Press, Inc., 2001, pp. 103-109.

The above assumption implies that one should proceed from the general to the specific. Accordingly, I will delineate the relatively small number of criteria or elements of the good life for humans in general, and point out any special implications to retarded people. However, in order to comprehend the following discussion, readers should keep in mind that mental retardation generally implies not only a deficit in intellect, and therefore also in judgment, but almost always also one in volition (see Wolfensberger, 1982), including, quite commonly, deficits in curiosity, initiative and self direction and usually also in other domains of identity, including personality.

THE ELEMENTS OF THE GOOD LIFE
FOR RETARDED PERSONS

God's Grace to Turn to Him

The first element of the good life for anyone must come entirely from God, and consists of the grace which enables a soul to choose God. Elsewhere (Wolfensberger, 1982), I have elaborated on the idea that even the souls of the most profoundly retarded persons probably make such a fundamental choice, and probably do so in this life. Assuming that this speculative assumption is valid, then it is very difficult from a Christian perspective to conceptualize a good life for a retarded person if that person's soul has set itself adamantly against God.

Mentally retarded people are highly likely to be devalued in and by the world, to be rejected, and to have all sorts of bad things done to them–indeed, to be brutalized and even deprived of life. They share this experience with many other devalued groups, though many of these others are less devalued and/or have more defenses. Paradoxically, this reality can actually be conducive to access to the good life.

While sentimental romanticizing about retarded people being "holy innocents" must be rejected, the truth is that by reason of their devalued identity, retarded people are apt to develop fewer of those attachments and securities in life that commonly become idols to other people: possessions, objects, money, national pride, weapons, buildings, artifacts, one's employer and/or employing organization, and so on.

Relatedly, retarded people's very impairment in ability to relate to the long-term future so often frees them from the false hopes and idolatrous commitments of the mighty of the world. Thus, they are less likely to be resistive to God's grace–but they are, nevertheless, profoundly dependent upon others for those structures that are conducive to spiritual growth and spiritual life. Most mentally retarded persons are very limited in their capacity and power to structure the physical and social environment around them. Yet this structure can be crucial to a retarded person's life conditions, life style, schedules and routines, associations, and mental and spiritual dispositions. This is where the next point becomes important.

The Mediation of the Presence of God Through Others

Once the soul of a retarded person is receptive to God, the good life for him/her is promoted through the formation of an explicit faith, and the nurturance of the person's gifts of the Holy Spirit. However, I propose that the single biggest impetus in that direction (for everyone, but especially so for a retarded person) is to have in one's life the benefit of supportive relationships of persons who (a) can influence a retarded person's life structures so that these become at the very least enabling, and preferably promoting, of the person's spiritual life and expression of spiritual gifts, and who (b) mediate the presence of God.

In most cases, the good life would at least in part be contingent on these relationships being with individuals who play major and significant roles in the person's life (close family members, close friends, teachers, supervisors, spiritual guides, etc.), and especially whose relationships with the person are of a long-term nature. This proviso is important when one considers that there may very well be persons, perhaps even in large numbers, who mediate the presence of God in a retarded individual's life, but who do so in relatively minor, intermittent, or fleeting relationships. Examples might be neighbors with whom one has only occasional contact, or some members of one's local congregation with whom one may not even have close contact every Sunday.

The importance of the mediation of the presence of God is poorly appreciated by many people who, instead, often place inordinate emphasis on catechesis, i.e., on relatively formal religious instruction which is essentially aimed at the intellect, despite the concrete media that may be employed because the catechumens are children or retarded.

Relatedly, because the ultimate emphasis is intellectual, insufficient importance is often given to the spiritual identity of the religious instructor(s). Instead, what are accepted or sought as sufficient criteria to be such an instructor are willingness to function as a teacher, some intellectual mastery of the subject matter, skilled use of media, or even only the ability to teach in a manner which is perceived to be particularly suitable for retarded persons–though in reality, exactly the opposite may be true.

In contrast to these approaches, I have observed that retarded people have shown the greatest spiritual growth if they are surrounded by Christians who are intently focused on their own personal and communal quest for holiness. Even among these, some have much more marked gifts of mediating the presence of God than others, and if such mediation takes place in the presence of a retarded person whose soul is receptive to God, then startling manifestations of the spirituality of the person can develop, including manifestations which I call "fall-transcending," i.e., which are outside ("above") the world of natural law and which are fractional anticipations of the identity and functioning of humans in their "extra-fallen" identity, their state prior to the fall, and after the restoration of all things.

The significant presence of God-mediating persons in the life of a retarded individual can be so powerful as to surpass anything achievable through any other medium, including through various explicit forms of religious instruction. That this is so becomes apparent over and over when retarded persons are interrogated in regard to the faith. Those who have experienced what one might call naturalistic forms of religious instruction will give relatively rote or even inappropriate replies. Those whose spirituality has developed through contact with persons who mediate the presence of God often give startlingly creative replies which suddenly turn the inquisitor into an awed, open-mouthed pupil of the kingdom of God.

Valued Membership in a Christian Communality

Conceivably, some of the above things might be present in the life of a mentally retarded person, but the person might nevertheless not be a member of a communal body, or if a member, perhaps only of a family. Therefore, I now stipulate that the third major element of the good life is valued membership in a Christian communal body. The communality I mean is ordinarily not one of, or primarily for, handicapped people, but of Christians in general who will assimilate a proportion of handicapped persons as members. By the very nature of communalities, both the membership of the person, and the communality itself, need to be relatively long-term ones. For many members, it may be life-long.

Communal membership is of the greatest importance to anybody, but assumes some additional importance for retarded persons, for the following reasons:

1. Even more than other people, retarded persons, by the very fact that they are retarded, are limited in their functioning and generally cannot stand alone. The supports of family or individual friends may go a long way to enable such a person to function, but they often are not sufficient to overcome the isolation and restriction in life experiences which the retarded person typically experiences.

2. Unless a communality is self-segregating or otherwise very inward centered, it usually affords great stimulation to its members, because communalities typically have a diverse membership and can offer many opportunities for involvement and participation in the world.

3. Communality provides greater continuity of relationship, guidance and protection for a mentally retarded person than do individual relationships that are not held together by some other bond. To the life of a mentally retarded

person, the death of parents, a guardian, a strong citizen advocate, etc., can be devastating. However, within a communality, there are so many and such overlapping relationships that a mentally retarded member would not be as greatly dependent upon any one other individual member. This is likely to be the case because different members may have played a great variety of roles in the person's life, whereas an individual such as a parent often combines in his/her person many roles, such as teacher, guide, moral conscience, director, friend, instrumental advisor or even decision maker, and expressive (affectional) supporter. Furthermore, within the communality, some members may be able to assume roles that may be difficult or impossible for many persons outside of a communality to establish. For instance, a parent can hardly take on the identity of a sibling, but within a communality, there may be a number of persons who might assume the role of an older or younger sibling to a retarded person, and thus fill some important needs.

4. Membership in a non-Christian social body or communality is good, but not good enough; there also needs to be valued membership, and in a Christian communality. Valued membership is much more likely to be attained by societally devalued people if they belong to a communal body–and especially a Christian communal one–than to other bodies. However, it should not be taken for granted that even a Christian communality will automatically and at all times value any retarded member. Much consciousness and effort to that end need to be taught and practiced.

Abundant Participation in the Human Experience

Ordinarily, communal membership implies a wide range of participation. However, such participation may be limited to the communality itself, or may be narrow for other reasons. Thus, I must specifically stipulate a fourth major element of the good life, namely, abundant participation in the human experience–hopefully as a part of, derived from, or backed up by, the person's membership in a Christian communality.

Participation means many things. One of these is integration, i.e., being physically and socially a part of things, even of the mundane routines of society, rather than being physically segregated, kept apart from culturally normative experiences, places and events, being excessively grouped with other people who are themselves on the margins of society or rejected by it, or being unnecessarily protected. Participation also includes a sharing in the universal experiences and struggles of the human race, the joys which may derive therefrom, as well as the sufferings. For most people, these joys would also include moments of rapture. Furthermore, from the very fact that the person would hopefully participate from a communal base, the person would be cherished, and therefore the experience of suffering would not be the result of abuse. But in the context of the faith, and with communal support, even the suffering experiences would have their elements of "triumph."

Participation also means encouragement and opportunities to exercise one's charismatic gifts, i.e., the gifts of the Holy Spirit, and to minister unto others, including, of course, to non-handicapped people.

However, participation can be severely constrained by afflictions of mind and body. Therefore, such participation needs to be prepared for, enabled and facilitated. This can be done by (a) nurturing the retarded person's faculties and talents–those of soul, body, senses, intellect, personality, etc., and (b) by assisting those who are the likely participants with the retarded person, such as members of a communality. Too many people hold the attitude that if a person is going to be retarded anyway, then it makes little difference how far they develop. This attitude is wrong; it denies retarded persons their actualization toward their God-given potential.

Indeed, it is part of the good life to be surrounded by people who have positive growth expectations for one, and a commitment to help one grow. Because of their vulnerability, retarded persons, even more than others, need a delicate balance among developmental challenge, kindness, and spiritual nurture in order to unfold their talents and spirituality and–if they are Christians–to practice their charismatic gifts.

A Good Christian Death

Finally, the good life for retarded persons would also include a good death, i.e., a reconciled Christian death. If a person is too retarded to have much religious awareness, the members of his/her communality would do the same as they might do for a non-retarded member who had become demented: i.e., offer prayer and worship at the person's side, pray for the person elsewhere and especially in communal worship, and observe the person's death with both mourning for their loss and joy for the member's entrance into eternal life and the presence of God.

CONCLUSION

Above, we emphasized the role played by various physical, social and religious structures in the spiritual life of retarded persons. It would be a mistake to trivialize, or even underestimate, their importance–or to interpret them as always decisive. Experience has revealed that an oppressive social environment can severely limit the spiritual life of a retarded person, whereas a liberating Christian environment can permit a most wondrous unfolding of a retarded person's spiritual life and charismatic gifts. However, one can also encounter retarded persons who had been severely deprived, brutalized, and not exposed to "naturalistic" religious instructions, but who have entered into an intimate discipleship with God once even only modest supports were made available to them. Such a phenomenon may very well be an instance of "God's freedom" (Brueggemann) to transcend the rational world, and to manifest Himself powerfully within it. At any rate, God is unlikely to deal severely with a person whose spiritual life has been stunted by the fault of others. To the contrary. "Judgment is stern for the exalted [but] the lowly may be pardoned out of mercy" (Wisdom 6:5-6).

Contemplating the five major points above, one may be struck by their parsimony. A critical reader of an earlier draft of this essay commented that some people might say: "Is this all there is to the good life for retarded persons?" There are always so many more ways to do something wrong than right that one is often astonished at how sparse truths may be as compared to their subversions. The above critic concluded, "Yes, this seems to be all there is-as far as it goes," meaning that it was hard for him to add any points, though any of the points itself could be greatly enlarged.

REFERENCE

Wolfensberger, W. (1982). An attempt to gain a better understanding from a Christian perspective of what "mental retardation" is. *National Apostolate with Mentally Retarded Persons Quarterly, 13*(3), 2-7.

The Normative Lack
of Christian Communality
in Local Congregations
as the Central Obstacle
to a Proper Relationship
with Needy Members

Wolf Wolfensberger, PhD

"The community of believers was of one heart and mind, and no one claimed that any of his possessions was his own, but they had everything in common. With great power the apostles bore witness to the resurrection of the Lord Jesus, and great favor was accorded them all. There was no needy person among them, for those who owned property or houses would sell them, bring the proceeds of the sale, and put them at the feet of the apostles, and they were distributed to each according to need" (Acts 4:32-35).

During the course of my life-long pilgrimage as a Catholic Christian, I kept making one discovery after another about the Kingdom of God. Some of these were merely the products of an open-minded search, others I attribute to the grace of God. It was only around 1980 that I gained the insight that the practice of communality–of which Acts 4:32-35 is one example–was not just

This article is an edited version of a lecture by the same title given on 27 May 1992 to the Religion Subdivision at the 116th annual convention of the American Association on Mental Retardation in New Orleans, LA.

The author would like to thank to Ruth Abrahams, Peter King, Ann O'Connor, Susan Thomas and Chris Welter for critical comments on an earlier draft of this manuscript. The author is also indebted to Dennis Schurter for drawing to his attention an article by Bailey (1993).

[Haworth co-indexing entry note]: "The Normative Lack of Christian Communality in Local Congregations as the Central Obstacle to a Proper Relationship with Needy Members." Wolfensberger, Wolf. Co-published simultaneously in *Journal of Religion, Disability & Health* (The Haworth Pastoral Press, an imprint of The Haworth Press, Inc.) Vol. 4, No. 2/3, 2001, pp. 111-126; and: *The Theological Voice of Wolf Wolfensberger* (ed: William C. Gaventa, and David L. Coulter) The Haworth Pastoral Press, an imprint of The Haworth Press, Inc., 2001, pp. 111-126. Single or multiple copies of this article are available for a fee from The Haworth Document Delivery Service [1-800-342-9678, 9:00 a.m. - 5:00 p.m. (EST). E-mail address: getinfo@haworthpressinc.com].

a nice thing if one could find it, but that it was Christ's intent that His disciples should live out the Christian faith in a communal fashion–in what I call Christian communality.

Over time, I also learned that many people have very faulty notions of what either Christian or non-Christian communality is, and this context does not allow an adequate exposition of it. Be it only briefly noted here that there are both secular and religious communalities. Either can be likened to a closely-knit extended family that cultivates close intercommunication, that hangs in together through thick and thin, where everybody helps everybody else, where members take care of their own and protect and defend any of their members who get into trouble with the larger world, where members put up with each other's shortcomings, and where these shortcomings are accepted or dealt with within the group.

In practice, communality is rarely total. Usually, it takes a range of forms between minimal to radical. However, for the moment, let us speak as if it were a unitary entity.

Secular communalities usually only manage to hold together by one of three bonds: (a) kinship; (b) an ideal, in which case it often functions as if it were a religion, even if it is not interpreted that way; or (c) necessity. As regards the latter, some stable rural communities can serve as examples. People in them may function interrelatedly even if there are neither strong bonds of idealism or affection, nor much kinship. Instead, people behave at least somewhat communally because they know that in the long run, no one is likely to make it on their own.

Communality based on religious or strong quasi-religious ideologies usually adds further elements of interpretation about how communality should be practiced. Such quasi-religious or religious communalities can be very intense, but are at risk of being split by religious or ideological issues, as exemplified by the long history of endless splits among the communal anabaptist groups.

Here, we are not only speaking about religious communality, but about Christian religious communality; and what that adds to religious communality generally will depend on how one perceives, and lives out, Christianity. Of great help to me in understanding Christian communality, and Christ's intent that His disciples practice it, has been a book by Gerhard Lohfink (1984), entitled *Jesus and Community,* also elaborated on by Bailey (1993).

Here is what Christian communality seems to imply to me. First, one does the things that generic communalities would do, and the family analogue of communality implies commitment to each other. But in addition, one does these things in the context of a life of Christian faith and worship. Thirdly, one does these things in a fashion that ties one's social behavior systematically to Christian rationales. Fourthly, on top of all this come the gifts and promises that pertain not to individual Christians, but to Christians who come together, are together, and stay together in Christ's name. The Lord would bring together people who complement each other, not only in natural talents, but also in gifts of the Holy Spirit. Additionally, He would bestow gifts, graces, and natural resources so that no member would be in want. On top of individual gifts of discernment would come a gift for collective discernment, which is quite different. Worship will display what I call fall-transcending manifestations–as, for instance, music and song that seem to come straight from heaven. The miraculous–which is also no more than fall-transcendence–will be commonplace, though usually not at all spectacular.

Indeed, there are some of us who believe that the dearth of miracles in Christianity after the fourth century is the result of two things: a turning away from radical nonviolence once Christianity allied itself with secular authority, and a retreat from communality.

Notions of Christian communality have not thrived within the Catholic parish structure, but at least two other traditions within Catholicism have kept notions of such communality alive: monasticism, and the innumerable local (and the fewer supra-local) confraternities in the Middle Ages, especially in the cities.

In Protestantism, Christian communality depended entirely on the respective local congregations. Communality there has tended to be more active than in Catholic parish life, but rarely anywhere near what I see as Christ's intent. The closest to it seem to be some of the radical dissidents from Catholicism in the pre-Reformation and early post-Reformation era, and significant sectors of the anabaptist movement since then.

Precisely because divine promises and empowerments go with Christian communality but not with non-Christian communality, Christian communality should be able to be even more radical than that of extended families, in terms of taking care of the needs of members.

It seems to me that one of the most fundamental questions before Christians comes down to this: do you believe that Christ intended Christian communality to be the normative way of living for His disciples? The answer to this question will divide Christians profoundly–in some respects as profoundly as issues such as the apostolic succession. It will determine how one perceives and interprets congregational life and congregational organization, property, evangelization, and how one should relate to needy or impaired Christians.

If one does not believe that Christian communality is the intended normative Christian life, then one will have to explain what all the New Testament passages that exhort to communality, or that exalt it, are supposed to communicate, or why they do not apply.

The next painful point is that there are hardly any local Christian church congregations that are communal. After counting the few residential congregations that are, in fact, communal (such as the Hutterites), probably the next highest proportion of communal congregations is among the other ana-baptists and maybe among charismatic communities; then there is a sprin-kling among the evangelicals, and then next to nothing among the "higher" or mainline denominations. Personally, I do not know of a single Catholic parish that functions communally. Rural churches often have at least more communal elements, even though few of them would qualify as truly com-munal.

Now I will deliver myself–so to speak–of a devastating opinion, namely, that most pastors do not present orthodox Christian teaching on Christian communality, and that they do not do so for the following five reasons.

1. Many simply do not know that this is supposed to be Christian ortho-doxy, and mostly they do not know because it has not been taught to *them*.

2. Most of them know that if they taught this truth, the message would be largely rejected, they themselves would be rejected, and they would not have a formal pastorate.

3. Many have embraced a most unChristian numbers game mentality. They believe in the merits of large memberships: not disciples, not holiness, not fall-transcending manifestations, not miracles, but numbers, and whatev-er will bring these in. After all, at least in part for the sake of numbers, Christians condone militarism, war, violence, sexual sins, homosexual be-havior, abortion, "euthanasia," and religious services based on Mickey Mouse, Peanuts and clown themes that open the door to dangerous influences from a media-possessed non-Christian pop culture–one often viewed by con-temporary Christians as superior to historical Christian culture. Anything that Christian individuals or bodies do that is unduly motivated by numbers–ori-ented calculations strongly suggests the dominance of two mindsets. (a) One does not believe that disciples will always be few in numbers. (b) One does believe that one's own fallen efforts will work conversions in those upon whom these efforts impinge, rather than that God will work them.

Particularly where a numbers game mentality prevails, calls for more radical communality are apt to be condescendingly interpreted as "impracti-cal," and greeted with admonitions to be "sensible" instead, much as one would hear in politics, the marketplace, finance, etc. But the bitter irony in all this is that when Christian denominations go for numbers, the long-term effect so often is *loss* of numbers–even among the merely casual members for whose sake so many accommodations have been made.

4. The numbers game mentality must not be confused with the fourth reason why pastors do not teach properly about Christian communality, namely, a modernistic exaltation of a "politically correct" construct of "in-clusiveness" in Christian circles, which means that anyone who wants to belong should be welcomed, regardless of what they either believe or do.

This saccharine–and certainly most unbiblical–inclusivity mentality is incompatible with communality, because communalities need to be extremely exclusive in order to become or remain communal.

5. Wherever there is imperiality of structure and style (such as spelled out best by the writings of Walter Brueggemann), true communality is a profound threat, for too many reasons that I cannot cover here. So in some church sectors, one encounters a mixture of deep fear, and even hatred, of communality. The very existence of communality would be perceived–and correctly so–as a critique of the prevailing imperiality, and as a threat to it.

Here is an example. The choir of a Catholic church in Evansville, Indiana, included a paraplegic singer, and in a true manifestation of Christian communality, the members of the choir carried this person up 18 steps to the choir loft every time they sang. Then somebody thought that this was too dangerous and complained all the way up to the bishop. The choir members began to raise money for an elevator, but the parish members voted against it. The choir would not give up its handicapped member, and so the pastor disbanded the choir with the approval of the bishop (AP in *Indianapolis Star*, 3 Feb. 90).

Here is an even more striking example. In 1992, Catholic authorities in the United States came down very hard on some charismatic communities. The directives that came down from above were of the kind that would not only address certain real problems and occasional excesses in charismatic communities, but would also make communality de facto impermissible. Some of these directives would make it impossible for a Catholic group to live a devout communal life in, but not of, a world that has embraced the overpowering values and lifestyles of modernism. So I interpret this crack-down to be directed more at communality than at excesses of pentecostal Catholicism–after all, *There has not been a public revelation of one single comparable crackdown by the hierarchy in all of North America against the excesses, and outright heresies and perversions, of the modernistic liberal Catholic left* (as of the date of this presentation, 1992).

Lohfink (1984) goes so far as to assert that the new covenant between Christ and His disciples is that if they are communal (e.g., "a new commandment I give you, that you love one another," John 13:34), and constitute what Lohfink (1984) calls a "divine contrast society," then God will do everything that this communality and its individual members need. If you do not believe this after reading the Bible, then read Lohfink!

In a commentary on both the Sermon on the Mount and Lohfink, Bailey (1993) makes the additional point that a Christian communality lives in a way that "would not make sense if a gracious God did not exist." He also interprets the New Testament scripture passages that point toward communality by disciples as being not a "law to be obeyed but a way of living rooted in the divine graciousness . . ." I would put it that it is Christ's will, which is not always a law. Many Christians are very confused about the difference, about which so much could be said.

Bailey (1993) also points out some of the reasons why Christ would want His disciples to live in Christian communality.

1. It maintains an eschatological vision. To this, I would add that it is obvious how easily such a vision is lost, especially in a context of a materialistic, here-and-now-istic, skeptical modernism. Also, such a vision supports hope within the worst imaginable events in the world.

2. Christian communality makes it more likely that one lives "poor in spirit."

3. A Christian communality that lives as a contrast society is more apt to be able to focus on God's righteousness, and thus put and keep things in right relationship to each other.

4. In Christian communality, there is both pain and joy, and because of the joy, the pain can be borne. This also averts the apathy and blunting of passion that is so normatively engendered by imperial powers.

Based on his conclusion that God will do what is needed for Christians who live communally, Lohfink (1984) calls into question the major prevailing models of evangelization–and above all, media evangelization–because they are either not based on, or not manifested by, communality. Lohfink says that the normative model of evangelization should be to live in radical Christian community, like the early Church did, and that hardly anything else is necessary, because the Lord will then work the miracles and the conversions in those who observe the living-out of communal discipleship. It will not be the preaching, teaching, audiovisuals, fancy music, clapping, or whatever, that will work the conversions. After all, note how in Acts 4, one of the two passages (v. 32) that inform us of the unity and sharing of the community of believers is immediately followed (v. 33) by one that tells us that the apostles bore witness "with great power," implying a cause-effect relationship. In the other parallel passage (Acts 2:42-47), verse 42 says, "They devoted themselves . . . to the communal life . . . ," and in verse 43, ". . . and many wonders and signs were done through the apostles"–again, as if the latter was a fruit of the former. Thus, Christian identity, especially as manifested in Christian communality, *is* mission (Bailey, 1993) more than any number of other things are.

One of the most decisive reform movements in Christianity–at least Western Christianity–was the Cluniac movement. It flowed from the establishment of the monastery of Cluny in France in 910. At this monastery, the monks were *not* to be primarily missionaries and teachers, but men living a life of prayer and sacred song in community. They engaged in *less* manual labor than other monks of their time, and their daily divine office was longer than that of the other monasteries. Yet out of Cluny came a reform that positively affected not only Western monasticism (with 1500 monasteries eventually being founded out of Cluny and its "daughter" monasteries), but the entire Western church. Today, people would say that all this happened despite the fact that Cluny "did nothing," rather than that it happened *because* Cluny did what people these days consider to be "nothing."

Now note how embarrassing–or even indicting–an assertion such as Lohfink's is. There are denominations these days that will do virtually anything to bring in the infidel–*except* practice Christian communality. They will hire expensive anti-Christian media firms,[1] harangue from television, try to make people feel good, promise forgiveness for unrepented sins, and on and on–and their numbers keep shrinking. Thank goodness!

The idea that conversion is largely a fruit of holiness, rather than the result of an evangelizing busybody "doing," is also underlined by the common historical phenomenon that nothing makes faith flourish more than persecution and martyrdom. No preaching or teaching or running medical services or tent revivals–just get persecuted or even killed for the faith, and true conversions drop like apples from the trees, and church is once more like in the days of Acts.

An example is Peter Chanel (1803-1841) who went to missionize Oceania, but had nothing to show for it after four years, and the mission seemed like a complete failure. Then he had one single very significant convert: the chief's son. This enraged the chief, who had Peter clubbed to death and carved up, making him the first Catholic martyr of Oceania–and within one year, the whole island had become Christian!

Had the media evangelists in the United States that have been brought to such shame in recent years been members of radical Christian communalities, many problems would have been prevented. Those who were phony to begin with would have been stopped by their communities. Those who started out properly but eventually waxed greedy would have been stopped at that point. Those who fell into habitual sexual sins might have been saved from these by the affection that is commonly exchanged among members of communalities, and/or by admonitions from the elders.

This concludes part one of my presentation, and I will now turn more specifically to implications to inclusion of handicapped and other needy people.

If one does not believe that Christian communality should be the norm in local congregations, then one obviously would have no motive for pursuing it. And if a Christian congregation does not want to pursue communality, then what might be its stance vis-à-vis handicapped or dependent people?

First of all, we have a very problematic situation where congregations are so constituted in the first place as to be virtually cut off from needy, poor, wounded, or dependent people, and this is certainly the case where the congregation has no–or virtually no–such people as members. On the one hand, congregations are in trouble if they have a disproportionately large number of such members, because then, the capacity of the other members to meet their needs would be overwhelmed. But it is a great sign of danger when a congregation has nowhere near what one might call an "expected" number of such members, particularly in a society where such people are plentiful. Such a congregation is apt to be one that is cut off from the suffering Christ–which, in my opinion, puts one's salvation at terrible risk. And such a lack of needy people in one's own congregation cannot be compensated for by "long-distance" charitable work, such as contributing to organized charities, or sponsoring overseas missions.

Aside from this issue, here are some of the things that one commonly sees done by Christian congregations vis-à-vis handicapped people, and perhaps other needy ones too.

1. Making physical facilities handicap-friendly, as with ramps.

2. Accepting needy people–especially for worship–but otherwise paying little attention to them.

3. "Integrating" needy people as members, but not communally.

4. Establishing "special ministries" for handicapped or minority groups, either on the congregational or higher level.

5. Rendering informal services to needy *non*-members, but not necessarily to needy members. For instance, members may give alms directly to needy non-members, or they may help out sick or impaired neighbors who are not members–all this while the needs of their fellow members are not addressed.

6. Employing non-members, and even non-believers, to run formal services, often even segregated ones, usually primarily to non-members. For instance, a church may hire an outreach worker who is not a member, or not even a believer. Such a person may even serve mostly non-members. Catholic parish schools may hire people–including non-believing non-members–to function as teachers (perhaps to a segregated class), and as many as the majority of the children may not belong to members, or even believers. Supra-congregational organizations are particularly apt to do such things, and to render services to handicapped people in segregated groups. A diocesan Catholic Charities agency may hire someone who is a member of a pagan witch cult to render social and relief services that are totally undistinguished (and undistinguishable) from those that would be rendered by a governmental office, or by a secular private agency, and without regard to whether the needs of the diocese's members get addressed.

In some of the cases above, and in some of the points yet to come, there may even be denial of the existence of handicapped members in one's flock. For example, I have so often heard of instances where pastors, when asked how many retarded people were in their congregations, said "none"–sometimes even after parents of retarded children had shared with the self-same pastor their problems and needs, and asked for help.

7. Seeking and accepting subsidies from Caesar to do any of the above.

8. Directing needy members for help to government, and other public and private service agencies, rather than to the congregation.

9. Sending money elsewhere to help out there, while members' needs are not met.

10. Playing up "peace and justice" themes, perhaps in relation to events far away, again while issues of violence and justice to one's own needy members go unaddressed.

11. Recruiting support for political candidates who support a church social agenda.

12. Doing things that bring in and retain needy people as members, regardless whether these (a) are believing Christians, (b) have a clear sense of their denominational identity, (c) are glad to be members, or (d) live in a way that reflects their faith.

I will now selectively elaborate on some of these points–mostly on Nos. 1 and 3, as well as some of the things that Christian communality would imply in reference to impaired or dependent persons.

A noncommunal congregation can be said to have members, though it may be difficult to tell apart those who are members and those who just "go to church there." Therefore, handicapped and dependent persons may be as much or as little integrated into such a church as nonimpaired members or attendees are. Yet such "integration" may be proclaimed pridefully as a great achievement.

If we come to believe in, and understand, the imperative for Christian communality, we can begin to see the limitations–and even insufficiencies–of what would generally be understood as "integration" in today's parlance. Most of what goes under the term "integration" is secular technology. Such technology can be not only material in nature (ramps, electronic sound amplification, elevators with beepers, etc.), but also social (manipulating people into togetherness, playing get-acquainted games, etc.). At the very least, such secular technology must never be deployed *in lieu of* Christian conduct, and above all, not in lieu of fall-transcending Christian practice. Some should never be practiced at all because it is tainted by its non-Christian or even anti-Christian origins or accompanying meanings.

Even where, in theory, it would be quite permissible to use various technologies that enable impaired persons to participate in a local congregation, in actual practice, the timing of the institution of such technological resources is very likely to have vast consequences. Namely, if the technologies are installed *before* a Christian resolution of communality has been achieved, then the technology is almost certain to displace–perhaps even prevent–such a Christian resolution. On the other hand, if a Christian resolution of communality is worked out first, the technology could be the icing on the cake–or could even turn out not to be very important anymore.

Communal membership, and particularly Christian communality, overlaps with integration, but is by no means identical to it. For instance, in the transaction of Christian communality, there would be an active interchange among all the elements of identity of the members. This means not only that natural talents and spiritual gifts would be employed in a fashion that is complementary among members, but that the weaknesses, shortcomings, and afflictions would be similarly exchanged and, in a sense, mutually complemented. For instance, the spiritual gifts of each member who is a disciple would be used by that member for the benefit of some, or even all, others. At the same time, members would also take on and bear with each other's afflictions and shortcomings. Thus, one of the processes of healing would be that the pains and sufferings of one member also become the sufferings, and possibly the pains, of one or more others. Obviously, one hears relatively little of this aspect of mutuality in the vast background of contemporary talk about "integration" or "inclusion."

Furthermore, the contemporary secular mentality has profound difficulties in saying anything positive not only about suffering itself, but also about human afflictions in general, and it commonly even denies that there *can* be anything positive about these. My knowledge of this was certainly reinforced when I published an article (Wolfensberger, 1988) in the April 1988 issue of *Mental Retardation* on some of the positive assets–as I called them, for lack of a better term–that are reasonably commonly found in retarded people. Even some of the ideologized people that one might call the "secular radicals" found many elements of this article very objectionable, or at the very least, discomfiting. For instance, some readers did not like my saying that retarded people are very often spontaneous and open in their affections, because saying so might play into stereotypes (e.g., of the happy and affectionate person with Down's syndrome), and because some retarded people are spontaneously affectionate in a way that violates normative societal customs. Some "secular radicals" also did not like my position that many retarded people have the capacity to engage in a single and/or simple activity for an extended period of time without becoming bored with it as a nonretarded person would (Wolfensberger, 1988, p. 67), because they did not like the implication that retarded people can be quite good at, and quite contented with, repetitive and even "menial" work. Thus, even some readers who had glimpses of the truths in this article did not like what they glimpsed.

The closest that members of the secular world come to voluntarily taking on the sufferings of the afflicted is through compassion, or by taking on some of the life conditions and roles of those people in society whom I call "the least"–and the latter does not happen very often.

How deeply the non-Christian secular modernistic attitudes toward suffering have crept into Christianity is brought out by the fact that so many individual Christians and Christian collectivities can no longer deal with the reality of a crucified Christ, but only a risen one–if they can deal with *any* divine Christ at all. This has been particularly dramatically manifested in Catholicism. Until the Second Vatican council, it may have dwelled too much on the suffering Christ, but in some Catholic contexts today, there simply is no longer a crucified Christ at all. Where formerly, one would have found images of the crucifixion, one now often finds images of the risen Christ, and the crucified Christ has been consigned to the trash–sometimes literally. The modernistic version of the Good Friday stations of the cross no longer ends with a meditation on Christ being laid in the tomb, but with Christ's resurrection–two days before it is observed liturgically on Easter! Modernistic Catholics cannot bear to watch with a suffering Christ for two days, but must have their feel-good now, even on Good Friday itself.

An interesting co-occurrence is that where Christians cannot deal adaptively with suffering, they usually also deny not merely that certain human acts constitute sin, but the very sinfulness of the human as well. Again, one of many spectacular manifestations of this is the virtual abolishment in some places or by some priests of the penitential rite at the beginning of the Catholic Mass. So commonly these days, this rite gets stripped of its penitential character, to the point where everything penitential about it is eliminated except the least and last vestige of reference to sinfulness that simply cannot be eliminated because of the liturgical rules.

One should not be surprised that where sinfulness cannot be acknowledged, suffering is almost certain to also be prettied up–and some kind of Enlightenment Christianity spreads out instead.

How does all this bear on Christian communality, and inclusion of afflicted people as members? First of all, the benefits of communality come at a high price–so high, in fact, that few Christians practice Christian communality. One of several such prices is that communality is painful, entails making many sacrifices (exemplified in Acts 4:34-35), much suffering, and requires confronting, dealing with, and also the sheer bearing of those sufferings that one could escape by escaping the communality. A second price is that one is confronted close up by the sins and sinfulness of fellow members. That is why a reductive explanation of communality is "putting up with each other." If one is unable or unwilling to do this, one cannot have communality. Unfortunately, within the context of a self-centered modernism, people normatively are encouraged from an early age *not* to "put up with" all sorts of things, and so they lack the disciplined habits of putting up even with their own family members, not to mention the demands of other communalities.

If one sees things the way I do, and has a bit of humor, one can say–scandalous as it might at first sound–that one of the worst things that ever happened to the inclusion of handicapped people in Christian church life was the invention of ramps. If congregations are really sophisticated, they may think that installing sound amplification for the hearing-impaired, or having a deaf interpreter, is the ultimate icing on the ramp cake. Yet ramps were perhaps the most clever means of the devil for *letting Christian congregations off the divine hook* (or, in the case of Catholics, out of the jaws of the hound of heaven) *as regards the expected practice of Christian communality.* Because this may seem so shocking a statement, I will now explain.

Ramps permit handicapped people to enter the church on their own, without either having to make any demands on other members, or without having to accept any help, and thereby also being able to avoid all sorts of social and physical contacts, and also a sense of dependence and indebtedness. This is not good for Christian communality. But in addition, ramps have done two other bad things. First, they give congregations the idea that they have done their duty, paid their dues, and have become an "affirmative congregation" (or whatever the current politically correct slogan may be) once they have installed a ramp. Second, ramps permit and enable handicapped people to be just as neutral, disengaged, individualistic and noncommunal participants as are the other participants–the ones who are able-boned, able-legged, able-hearing, able-sighted, able-hearted, etc. And yet, such achievements may be announced with considerable satisfaction as successful integration.

Of course, afflicted and handicapped people are just as much affected by the contemporary modernisms as anyone else, meaning that among Christian handicapped people, one finds the same demands and attitudes that one finds among the non-Christian–handicapped or nonhandicapped–people of the world. For instance, handicapped people commonly argue that it is the physical alteration to the church building that constitutes the enablement of church membership, and the willingness of a congregation to have these alterations made has become the touchstone of congregational political correctness.

Of course, I am *not* arguing against having ramps, but I am focusing very disproportionately on the ramp because it has become something like an icon–and a bad one at that: the single most visible symbol in people's minds of having done something for the handicapped in one's church. Not surprisingly, it is often also the ugliest part of the building.

But this kind of thinking is a very curse of modernism. I assure you–if you reflect on it just a bit you will know it is true–that there were full church memberships prior to the age of affluence and modernism; that there were people who were blind, deaf, lame, halt and crippled who were fully members of their braille-less, electronic-less and ramp-less churches. Yet one thing is for sure: the less communality such churches practiced, the less were the handicapped likely to be members–but the less were the *non*handicapped as well.

A handicapped Christian disciple would realize that, hard as it may be to bear, being physically carried into the church building (provided one is not dropped!) may be infinitely more valuable for literally everyone involved than having the church build a ramp. It is membership, and membership participation, that becomes the decisive criterion, not physical access, not accessibility, and not the attainment of legal rights. As part of the Christian communality, the afflicted person would strive to be, so to speak, graciously afflicted, and would accept certain hardships and problems that go with the affliction, while *also* being shamelessly aware of–and practicing–his or her gifts, and particularly those gifts or endowments that, for the benefit of others, may be linked to the very affliction itself.

Instructively relevant to the image of being carried into church is the following story. In 1991, two mountain climbers carried a paraplegic man up Yosemite Half Dome. It took them 13 days–and was not exactly necessary. However, the media interpreted the man who got carried up as a "climber"–a valued social role, and a good example of Social Role Valorization (Wolfensberger, 1983, 1992), even though the attribute was quite exaggerated. How little it would take to carry this man up a step or two into a church and call him a "member"–without exaggeration! In Acts 3:10, we learn of a physically handicapped man–very possibly with cerebral palsy, judging from Peter's special effort to have the man look at him–who was carried to the temple gate every day. In Christ's days, people were available aplenty to carry the handicapped about; and in one dramatic scene, they carried a man up onto a roof and lowered him by ropes in front of Christ, there to be healed (Matthew 9:1-8; Mark 2:1-12; Luke 5:17-26). But if the cripple had been a modernist, he would have insisted on getting to Christ in his own wheelcart or on those wooden blocks on which crippled people often moved about until modern days–and would probably not have been healed, but instead received many "rights," and a perverted sense of self-esteem and dignity.

Another difference between integration and the practice of Christian communality together with one's afflicted members is that the very afflictions can become the channel of those good things–including divine gifts and graces–that the community would otherwise lack. I am certainly not implying that God–rather than the demonic–is the source of sickness or handicap, but I do mean that the Lord may indeed bestow endowments and gifts on impaired people that will be exercised or expressed precisely *through and because of* their afflictions, rather than through some other part of the identity or experience of themselves or the other members. A prime example that should be familiar to all of us is the peculiar and striking truthfulness that some retarded people manifest precisely because of their concreteness of mind–a concreteness that is part and parcel of their mentally retarded condition, and that prevents them from engaging in the kind of denial or dressing up of truths that is so normative among smart people. Elsewhere (Wolfensberger, 1988), I have commented on this phenomenon at greater length, and on other positive behaviors sometimes displayed by retarded persons precisely by virtue of their retardation.

Just how corrupted the construct of integration can get even in a Christian context of great earnestness is underlined by two common contemporary phenomena.

1. Various bodies of Christians of great earnestness are bringing in experts to tell them how to do integration–even though these experts are not Christian, and may even be allied to great evils, such as various forms of death-making: abortion, euthanasia, capital punishment, war, lavish use of prescription psychoactive drugs, etc. Just what fruit do Christians think they can possibly get from this? (One person who critiqued an earlier draft of this article asked at this point, "Whatever happened to common sense?")

2. There are people (at least in North America) who are not Christian, who do not even belong to any explicit religious identity, but who are strongly involved in promoting integration of handicapped people into Christian churches as a purely secular psychosocial technology. With only minor hyperbole, whether the handicapped person gets integrated into a sex club, a pro-abortion group, a satanic cult or a Christian church is all the same to them, but Christian bodies permit such promoters to be their pace-setters, leaders, and consultants. Thereby, instead of being a light *to* the world (Matthew 5:14), they are following the lights *of* the world (to which one manuscript critic added, "and they will certainly live to rue the day").

By the way, one thing that all of this points to is that there is a real dearth of elaboration these days of what it would mean to be a handicapped disciple vis-à-vis contemporary modernism. It would be good to hear some deeply spiritual handicapped Christians shouting out to other Christians, both handicapped and nonhandicapped, "Stop! You've got it all wrong! You are caught up in the agendas of worldly modernism, not in the politics of Jesus and God's kingdom on earth." There are a few such voices,[2] but they do not get readily disseminated, they are more likely to be drowned out by the secular culture of political correctness of how one should be handicapped, and they are apt to be pilloried as traitors and Uncle Toms by the dominant modernistic handicap culture.

Contemporary modernistic Christianity is flawed by many very fundamental errors, and one of these is the assumption that religion rests on doing, rather than primarily being. Christianity implies first of all a submissive faith; secondly, a state that is, in fact, a form of inner doing but that is better talked about as being, and as being in goodness; and finally, a sphere of doing in the sense of overt action that is a derivative of faith and being, and that for most people is quite properly of very modest scope, since the first two things simply do not leave much time for doing anything else, especially if one also has to earn a living.

Lest I leave a wrong impression, let me emphasize a few things that I most emphatically do *not* understand to be expressions of Christian communality.

1. First of all, admission to a communality must be vastly more rigorous than processes of admission are today in the vast majority of churches. Being joined in communality is not the same as being joined in marriage, but it should have a similarity to it in terms of exploration, the testing during courtship, the last chance to reconsider during engagement, etc. The early church after the apostolic era had a very rigorous admissions process, probably in reaction to the indiscriminate admission during the apostolic era that, among other things, led to all sorts of perversions and squabbles even in apostolic days, as we can read in the epistles and the Book of Revelation.

2. Practice of Christian communality does not mean that one goes out and tries to drag in as a member every needy person one finds *because* they are needy. Instead, one takes care first and foremost of the needs that already exist, or arise, within one's membership. Also, whatever needy members one invites should meet the same criteria as other members in terms of repentance, desire of the soul, spirit of communality, etc. Some people who are dependents of full members may lack these prerequisites, and must be viewed as being different kinds of members–perhaps more like participants–toward whom one has obligations, but who do not hold offices, from whom one cannot demand full reciprocity, and who cannot participate fully in the communal discernment processes, if at all. Of course, such participants may, in time, grow into fuller membership.

3. It does not mean that one starts running services for needy non-members. One will be able to render a small amount of works of mercy in an informal fashion to non-members, but not much. The bulk of the efforts that are not devoted to earning a livelihood will be turned inwards. I consider it to be one of the great scandals of Christian churches that they take care of non-members while not taking care of their needy members.

There are many other common misconceptions about communality in general, and Christian communality specifically, which I cannot address here.

If I am right, then it follows that church leaders are in a terrible bind when it comes to the inclusion of handicapped people. If leaders taught that this inclusion must be part of Christian communality, and that in some cases it implies heroic actions, such as the congregation *informally* taking over the formal functions of the human service system vis-à-vis this or that needy member, then these leaders would be "on the outs" in most cases. If they promote "ramp integration," they are not fully honest, either to their congregations in general, nor to handicapped people specifically.

One of the ways one pastor explained away the model set by the early Church was in terms of the very modernistic argument that new is better than old, e.g., times are different now, and old ways are not necessarily better than new ones.

NOTES

1. An example is the Catholic bishops of America who in 1991 hired the Hill & Knowlton public relations firm in order to design a Catholic anti-abortion PR campaign–a firm that had designed advertising for oodles of God-less and deathmaking enterprises, including some for abortion.

2. An example is a short address (O'Connor, 1989) by a physically very handicapped member of the Christian–although admittedly very limited–communality to which I belong. It speaks at least somewhat to that issue.

REFERENCES

Bailey, J. L. (1993, March-April). Sermon on the Mount: Model for community. *Currents in Theology & Mission*, 85-94.

Lohfink, G. (1984). *Jesus and community: The social dimension of Christian faith.* (Trans. by J. P. Calvin). Philadelphia: Fortress Press; & New York: Paulist Press.

O'Connor, A. (1989, August). A few reflections on differentness. *Person to Person Citizen Advocacy Newsletter* (Syracuse, New York). Pp. 2-3.

Wolfensberger, W. (1983). Social Role Valorization: A new term for the principle of normalization. *Mental Retardation, 21*(6), 234-239.

Wolfensberger, W. (1988). Common assets of mentally retarded people that are commonly not acknowledged. *Mental Retardation, 26*(2), 63-70.

Wolfensberger, W. (1992). *A brief introduction to Social Role Valorization as a high-order concept for structuring human services.* (2nd (revised) ed.). Syracuse, NY: Training Institute for Human Service Planning, Leadership and Change Agentry (Syracuse University).

RESPONDERS

A Chaplain's Response

Dennis D. Schurter, DMin, BCC

The first time I heard of Dr. Wolf Wolfensberger was in 1978 when he made a presentation to the Religion Division at the AAMD annual meeting. I was a young chaplain at one of my first conventions. I spotted the poster in the hallway stating that he was a "distinguished lecturer." Because of the size of the crowd, the gathering was moved to a larger room, but the only one available was a restaurant area converted to an assembly hall. The room was packed. The lights were dim. But I found the edge of a table to sit on. I remember being impressed with the amount of information that he shared. But the enduring memory that I have carried through the years from that encounter was his discussion of people with mental retardation as the wounds in the body of Christ. When the Risen Christ reached out His hands to Thomas, he gave the invitation, "Touch my wounds and see and believe." Those with mental retardation and other disabilities are the wounded ones in the Body of Christ today. And today we are invited to touch His wounded ones and see and believe (cf. "An Attempt Toward a Theology . . .").

When Wolfensberger created this image in my mind, he seemed to speak a prophetic word to me–not in the sense of foretelling my future in ministry,

Dennis D. Schurter is Chaplain of the Denton State School, Denton, TX, and President of The Religion Division, AAMR.

[Haworth co-indexing entry note]: "A Chaplain's Response." Schurter, Dennis D. Co-published simultaneously in *Journal of Religion, Disability & Health* (The Haworth Pastoral Press, an imprint of The Haworth Press, Inc.) Vol. 4, No. 2/3, 2001, pp. 127-131; and: *The Theological Voice of Wolf Wolfensberger* (ed: William C. Gaventa, and David L. Coulter) The Haworth Pastoral Press, an imprint of The Haworth Press, Inc., 2001, pp. 127-131. Single or multiple copies of this article are available for a fee from The Haworth Document Delivery Service [1-800-342-9678, 9:00 a.m. - 5:00 p.m. (EST). E-mail address: getinfo@haworthpressinc.com].

although I have continued in my calling to serve people with mental retardation for most of my career–but in the sense of speaking a word from God that
touched my heart and that has in some way helped to undergird my ministry.
In responding to his articles, I want to point up what I see as Wolfensberger's
role as a prophetic voice for our age, for our faith communities, and for our
field of service to people with disabilities.

First, some observations concerning Wolfensberger's style and language
that might be considered characteristic of a prophet voice. His language and
style is filled with energy and enthusiasm, sometimes using extreme terminology to express his view and grab the reader's attention. He uses disturbing images of idolatrous materialism, church structures in defiance of the will
of God, and a haranguing style against "abortion, infanticide, and euthanasia." Through his language and style he sometimes seems to spew the passion of the prophet across the page. For me this is reminiscent of prophetic
figures such as Jeremiah, Hosea, Amos, and John the Baptizer. These are the
very characteristics that, at times, make me want to stop reading and fling his
papers aside. They are also the very things that urge me to think and consider
more deeply what he is saying. This is the role of a prophet.

Wolfensberger's prophetic voice speaks in several areas that I want to
highlight. First, he speaks forcefully concerning the fallen nature of our
world, our social structures, and our selves. This is certainly not a popular
message, nor is it one that is frequently heard. In the "Bible Belt" part of the
country where I live, this message usually focuses on the fallen nature of the
individual and one's personal need for God's salvation. But even here, one
hears little talk about the "fallen nature" of the social structures which make
up our local communities–the city council, the county commissioners, or the
local school board. Much less do those of us who are entwined in the social
service system or the educational structures of universities want to hear that
our own systems are "fallen" or corrupted or "gone bad" in some sense. We
choose to ignore such a message–and yet, we may find ourselves continually
frustrated by the ineffectiveness of our own efforts and the misguided direc-
tions of the systems we serve. Perhaps these are indications of the failing and
fallen nature of these systems. The fact that *we* serve the systems rather than
the other way around may also be indicative of some truth in his prophetic
voice.

Wolfensberger's emphasis on the idolatry of this modern age runs tandem
with the idea of the fallen creation. It is easy for me to identify with his
concern about the materialism of our culture and the many aspects of the
media that undermine our spirituality. On the other hand, his discussion of
technology gives me greater pause for thought. The capabilities given us by
computers and other technologies are playing an ever growing part in our
service systems for people with disabilities. Whole careers are built around

the new technologies and how to use them for the greater independence of individuals. Wolfensberger's warning here may be telling us that these modern miracles are not the keys to independence because they do not address our needs for nurture, love, and community. And he may be saying something more. Here again is a message that deserves our thoughtful ruminations.

A second prophetic word from Wolfensberger concerns the importance of community, or "communality," as he prefers to call it. (I use these two words interchangeably.) This is a theme that runs through all his papers, and with good reason since we are a culture that recognizes in a vague sense our need for community but has little sense of how to achieve it. The book *Habits of the Heart* by Robert Bellah and others validates Wolfensberger's pronouncements. Bellah's study is one example of a critique of the American culture that highlights our society's deep-seated individualism and our difficulties in achieving shared purpose and community.

Wolfensberger's five elements of the good life (cf. "The Good Life for Mentally Retarded Persons") have communality at their core. Communality happens to be element number three in the center of the list, but the importance of relationships and community are at the core of all five elements: (1) being open to God; (2) God mediated through others; (3) communality; (4) abundant participation in the human experience, clearly with other people; and (5) a good Christian death, not isolated from others, but valued by other people.

What makes Wolfensberger's words on community so provocative, even for me as a "professional in the field," is that he sets people with disabilities at the center of his call for communality. His idea is not only that people with mental retardation should be included in "our" communities, but that they can teach us about community and the power of sharing life together. This is not a new idea for me, but his words stir my heart and bring me up against concepts and realities that I tend to forget or ignore. And that is part of the power of the prophetic word.

These papers represent Wolfensberger's thinking and writing over a span of twenty years. Yet the message on community has not been heard by most of the faith communities who include ministry with people with disabilities. During the more than twenty years that I have worked with local congregations who have reached out to people with mental retardation, I have continued to struggle with them to actually integrate and include these adults with disabilities. In some of the congregations that I support as resource person, a few persons do the teaching and nurturing for that group of adults while the rest of the congregation does its best to ignore them. For years the rest of the congregation members may ignore pleas for friendship and inclusion and support for those who happen to have disabilities. The adults with disabilities are present in the congregation, but they are not part of the community. There is little sense of integration or communality. This may be a reflection of the lack of community within the congregation generally. If that's the case, this prophetic word is all the more important for the members and the leadership of the congregation to hear.

Wolfensberger highlights the L'Arche communities (cf. "The Prophetic Voice . . .") as examples of how people with mental and physical disabilities are calling others into community and helping all who will listen to know the power of supporting one another. The faith communities of our nation need to hear the power and message of this movement. Another person who has lived and spoken a similar prophetic word is Henri Nouwen. Through his personal struggle for direction, purpose, and calling in his life, Nouwen moved from the halls of academia at Yale through the Central American missions to the homes of adults with disabilities at the Daybreak Community in Toronto. After a lifetime of searching, he finally settled where he belonged, serving and growing in his relationships with those people who had special needs but who could also teach him special lessons about life.

One reason that Wolfensberger's message on communality strikes a chord with me is that I have spent most of my career as chaplain in a large residential facility (yes, an institution!). On the one hand, I have seen the sense of community that grows between those who live at the facility and some who work there. I have seen employees stay with low paying jobs because they truly care about the people who live there. But on the other hand, I have seen and experienced the isolation created by the institutional environment as those who live there are segregated from the larger community, just as Wolfensberger describes. I have seen many people who live there go through cycles of abandonment and grief through the decades of their lives. All of us who live and work at such a facility are a community, but we are a community isolated and set apart from the larger society. This larger society needs to hear and feel prophetic voices such as Wolfensberger's.

A third theme that is mostly implied in Wolfensberger's papers is a word to all of us who work as professionals serving people with mental disabilities. That theme states that we need to see ourselves first as people concerned about people and only secondarily as professionals using skills we have learned to help others. We must continually discern the reason that we entered the profession in the first place–if that reason revolves around the desire to nurture and care for others. The professional skills we have are simply tools to carry out that calling. The real power behind the professional person is the heart that has the desire to engage another person, to nurture the other person, and to learn with another person. As chaplains, physicians, educators, or social workers, we dare not lose touch with the heart of our calling which first propelled us into our work.

He makes this point when he talks about religious education, and thus religious educators, in "The Prophetic Voice and Presence . . . " He states, "Religious education is only a means, a technology towards a goal, not the goal itself." Thus, the tools and skills we claim as part of our respective professions are only a means to the end of service and wholeness for the people served. Service and wholeness only come when tools and skills help one heart touch another heart–when one person heals another. When that happens, it may be the person with a disability who is healed–and it may be the professional.

By way of a concluding reflection, it seems to me that when I read or hear the words of a prophetic voice, I may feel the urge to reject the message and the messenger. I may react strongly to his or her language and images which are disturbing. I may feel a threat to my sense of self as a professional. I may even hear a summons to change my way of thinking or acting. These may be the signs that I am hearing a prophetic voice.

I sometimes feel that way when reading Wolfensberger's writings. This is my response, for example, to his message about the power of evil in the institutional structures in which I have built my career. A fear arises within, and I fear to hear the challenge that he raises to my own work within the church structures and the institutional structures of my life. I feel a need to defend my position, my work, perhaps even the structures in which I have labored.

But a truly prophetic word will not only raise a challenge and a threat to my present way of life but will also offer a "way of escape" (I Cor. 10:13), a word of grace, a power that points beyond the past and present to the future. Wolfensberger's message does just that by pointing us to the very people whom we seek to serve, people with disabilities. They summon us back to the heart of our calling. They beacon us into community. They invite us to love and serve from the heart.

For these reasons I hope that church workers and leaders and professionals in all areas will read and consider what Wolfensberger has to say. We may disagree, we may argue, but we may also be touched and called and summoned to reconsider a path, a purpose, a direction in our lives.

The Works of Wolf Wolfensberger

Sandra L. Friedman, MD, MPH

As a developmental pediatrician, working in the field of Developmental Disabilities, I have been aware of Wolf Wolfensberger's pioneer work in normalization and social role valorization (Wolfensberger, 1983). As such, I admired his innovative way of thinking and stance against the prior social norm of segregation. While some of his writings had religious reference (Wolfensberger, 1988), I was not aware of his strong religious background, and its influence on his conceptualization of how individuals with mental retardation should live within the community, more specifically the Christian community. In reading the six articles dating from 1976 to 1992, I found nuggets of gold within the text of his writing. I admired his all-encompassing approach to those with mental retardation, and his criticism of perfunctory inclusion or guise of inclusion.

On the other hand, I had a difficult time following some of the logic he used to arrive at his conclusions, which in part may have been due to our different theological frameworks. Notwithstanding this different frame of reference, I found his articles to have elements of Christian elitism that at some level nourishes doctrines that incite prejudice in others. I found his intense distrust of science and technology to be rather parochial and short-sighted. I also found his conceptualization of those with mental retardation as representing prophecy to run counter to my views of the world.

While I do not consider myself to be "religious," I do believe that my Jewish heritage has had a profound impact on how I approach the world. It has always been important to treat all people, regardless of race, religion, socioeconomic status, or level of functioning, with respect and care. The

Sandra L. Friedman is Director of Pediatric Training, Institute for Community Inclusion/University Affiliated Program, Children's Hospital, Harvard Medical School, Boston, MA.

[Haworth co-indexing entry note]: "The Works of Wolf Wolfensberger." Friedman, Sandra L. Co-published simultaneously in *Journal of Religion, Disability & Health* (The Haworth Pastoral Press, an imprint of The Haworth Press, Inc.) Vol. 4, No. 2/3, 2001, pp. 133-138; and: *The Theological Voice of Wolf Wolfensberger* (ed: William C. Gaventa, and David L. Coulter) The Haworth Pastoral Press, an imprint of The Haworth Press, Inc., 2001, pp. 133-138. Single or multiple copies of this article are available for a fee from The Haworth Document Delivery Service [1-800-342-9678, 9:00 a.m. - 5:00 p.m. (EST). E-mail address: getinfo@haworthpressinc.com].

133

importance of helping those in need, community service, and opening one's home, are major underpinnings of the Jewish faith and of the concepts of "mitzvot" (blessings) and "tzedakah" (charity). Quite frankly, I never applied the concepts of the soul and Satan to my professional work, which were prominent features in the writings of Dr. Wolfensberger. Unlike Dr. Wolfensberger, I do not believe that affliction is the result of satanic forces. I believe that things happen irrespective of ancestral sin, that some things are not the result of Divine intervention, and free will does exist.

Dr. Wolfensberger's 1976 article, "The Moral Challenge of Mentally Retarded Persons to Human Services," suggested that increased visibility of people with mental retardation serves as a prophecy to herald in the collapse of society, and was reflective of the negative impact of intelligence with its associated science and technology. While I disagree with the preceding contention, I do agree with the importance of the development of informal relationships, genuinely shared worship and other activities.

He also forecasted the legalized destruction of those with severe disabilities. One may contend that the current debate on physician assisted suicide and euthanasia is consistent with this forecast. However, while those in need are at greatest risk of having their human rights infringed upon, this debate is occurring within the context of society in general, rather than in the disability community specifically (Meir, D., Emmons, C., Wallenstein, S., Quill, T., Morrison, R.S., Cassell, C., 1998). I do think that we need to be vigilant to prevent any abuses within the medical system, particularly towards those who cannot speak for themselves.

From a Jewish perspective, learning and knowledge have always been of great value. It is hard for me to accept that science and technology are directly responsible for the potential collapse of society. Rabbi Menachem Mendel Schneerson, an esteemed Jewish leader, has noted that science on its own is morally neutral, and technology, as with all forces, can be used constructively or destructively (Schneerson, M., 1995). I do believe that there is always a need to have ethical and moral guidelines, but to deny new knowledge and progress for fear of the unknown, only serves to keep one from unfolding the mysteries of the universe. One can believe in God and theological teachings, and still accept new, secular knowledge. In fact, the kabbalists' (Jewish mystical scholars) view is that science is a means to use the human intellect to obtain the truth, and that "both science and religion derives from the Source of all" (Sheinkin, 1986).

The article written in 1978, "An Attempt Toward a Theology of Social Integration of Devalued/Handicapped People," provided an interesting historical review of integration in early Christian society, particularly in the Middle Ages. While the communal approach to the infirm and those with disabilities was mentioned in a favorable light, I could not help myself from thinking about the persecution of the Jews and the violations of their human rights during that very same historical period. He spoke about the deleterious rise of segregation that occurred concurrently with the rise of intellect and science during the Renaissance, and progressed toward the end of the 19th century when "medicine abandoned its moral, philosophical, and theological background," and then peaked during the Nazi era. I agree that our society became more complex, with large variation in individual goals, experiences, and perspectives. Unfortunately, the increased complexity meant a more impersonal world. Religion does provide a framework for moral and ethical ways of living, however there are numerous historical examples of the very religious who were prejudiced, lacked compassion and acted immorally.

While nothing stays constant, social systems need to change to keep up with the times. All change is not bad; it is important to welcome knowledge and the change that it brings, striving toward changes that stand for the good of all. I agree that many of the changes of modernity have been negative, but that does not mean we should stop progress. Rather, we need to progress in a way that is morally and spiritually appropriate. I do wholeheartedly agree, however, that the rationale in support of integration significantly outweighs arguments in support of segregation.

"An Attempt to Gain a Better Understanding from a Christian Perspective of What "Mental Retardation" Is," written in 1982, was an article that was hard for me to digest. Again, our different theological perspective certainly impacted my impression of the article. This article spoke in detail about the human soul. Again, I had difficulty comprehending his contention that recognizing God, and then directing one's will away from God, can willfully cause one to be mentally retarded. While I disagreed with his concept of the fallen soul, and affliction being due to one's ancestor's sin, I did agree with the importance of love and inclusion.

The 1983 article, "The Most Urgent Issues Facing Us as Christians Concerned with Handicapped Persons Today," discusses signs of our time. He noted 17 signs of our time, which I will not enumerate here. However, I could not help feeling that while many of his concerns had valid underpinnings, there was a true fear for things that were new. He contended that the scientific advances put forth represented a lack of respect for moral authority, and that many in the medical profession have made "alliances with death." He acknowledged the complexity of science and technology. This increase in complexity was felt to be associated with decrease in human control and increase in demonic control. A fascination of the Eastern "cults" was felt to represent a repudiation of Judeo-Christian beliefs and a hedonistic utilitarianism. The signs noted were felt to portend the end of times, perhaps nuclear war. It was felt that because of human's intellectual arrogance, God was raising the importance of the "littlest" people, with individuals with mental retardation serving as prophets to an intellectually bankrupt world. He went on to cite a number of Christian responses to these signs, which were to reaffirm one's commitment to God and Creation, develop Christian alternatives to human services, and develop more personal and informal relationships with those with mental retardation.

Again, while some of his observations appeared to be on the mark, some extracted religious meaning to social change where I do not believe it exists. In many ways there has been a greater emphasis on moral and ethical issues as years have progressed. The issues of abortion and capital punishment are heated issues that will continue to be debated. However, these issues are not synonymous with a pervasive disrespect with human life at all levels. There have been many advances in humane treatment of patients in both the clinical and research fronts.

I believe that the turning toward Eastern religions seen in society often reflects the failure of religious teachings and way of family life. While Dr. Wolfensberger might contend those failures to be caused by science and technology, I think the relationship is more associative than causative. As one searches for greater meaning in life, young people may look outside their ken because of the belief that their own religion failed them, even though they may not have been adequately exposed to its doctrines. We live in a complex and pluralistic society. Progress brings wonderful benefits, but with those benefits come complexities that need to be addressed. The alternative would be to remain stagnant, which I believe runs counter to the human condition.

The other article written in 1983, "How We Carry the Ministry with Handicapped Persons to the Parish Level" addresses the need to know the relation between creation, the fall, redemption, and restoration. I certainly cannot address this concept with any authority from a theological perspective. The importance of Christian communality was discussed, with members supporting each other like an extended family. The concept of being accepting to community members is a good one, and one to be admired. I see this way of living as one alternative to providing a more accepting and loving environment. The concepts of family, community, and opening one's arms to others are important in the Jewish way of life. Belonging to a caring group is another way of acceptance of those with disabilities, and is a concept to be lauded. However, I believe that the group could be Muslim, Buddhist, Jewish, humanist, etc. I think the important issue is of belonging to a group with a common bond and being accepted as an individual with something to contribute to the whole. The group may have very strong ideological or theological underpinnings, but still should be one that respects all individuals and does not harbor the notion of supremacy of one group over another.

The last paper, entitled "The Normative Lack of Christian Communality in Local Congregations as the Central Obstacle to a Proper Relationship with Needy Members," was presented in 1992 at a meeting of the American Association on Mental Retardation. Dr. Wolfensberger noted that Christ intended his disciples to live in a communal manner, and thus communality is a way of living to which Christians should aspire in order to obtain Divine promises. He perceptively noted that many "easy" ways to accommodate those with disabilities allow people to feel more comfortable with their response without really acting to effectively include those with disabilities. I could understand the importance of having those with common Christian beliefs and values teach and work with the community, rather than having someone unfamiliar with the belief system. The unconditional acceptance of all members and the common bond of faith are important. However, I was struck with the theme of communality without ever a mention of family or the importance of family life. While the community may indeed act as an extended family, a person's nuclear and biological extended family needs to be acknowledged as the starting point for further outreach. He also mentioned that a person's "affliction" may provide the community with a channel for good things, and a person may express a gift from God through and because of his disability, even though the disability itself may be of demonic origin. I do not believe that a person's disability can be viewed as a gift of God or as a demonic expression. I believe those concepts only serve to set people apart rather than to bring them together, and perhaps reflect our need to have an explanation for everything even though one may not exist. There are some things that occur without fault and without being part of a larger scheme.

I was struck with the somewhat disparate need for integration of those with disabilities within a Christian community, while segregating the group from those who were not true believers or who do not abide by the concept of Christian communality. While a group needs to look after its own, we also live within a larger society that needs to be acknowledged. Again, my own theological background may be overshadowing this notion, as Jewish people do not have groups who live monastic lives apart from society as a whole. Rabbi Harold Kushner has noted that being Jewish is about finding a community. He speaks of the holiness of joining with other people, not fleeing imperfect neighbors to be alone with God (Kushner, 1993).

Through the years, Dr. Wolfensberger stayed true to the importance of integration, inclusion, and genuine acceptance of those with disabilities. The importance of every living being has also been an ever-present concept in his writings. I found him to become more exclusionary from a Christian standpoint, with the advancing chronology of his writings. Some of his observations were wake-up calls to evaluate social systems. However, I think that he had an unnecessarily alarmist approach to modern advances that were associated with negative social events, rather than the direct cause. Perhaps he would call me a liberal secular physician, or one that is not in the good graces of God because I am not Christian. While I admire his pioneer work in the field of mental retardation and community inclusion, I cannot accept his parochial view of the world. While Jews acknowledge their Biblical covenant with God, they believe that anyone can be close to God and achieve the highest spiritual state (Sheinkin, 1986). Unfortunately, history has revealed that attitudes of religious righteousness have often been responsible for pushing people apart rather than bringing them together.

REFERENCES

Kushner, H., (1993). *To Life.* Boston: Little, Brown, and Company.

Meier, D.E., Emmons, C., Wallenstein, S., Quill, T, Morrison, R.S., Cassell, C.K., (1998). A National Survey of Physician-Assisted Suicide and Euthanasia in the United States. *New England Journal of Medicine,* 338, 1193-1201.

Sheinkin, D., (1986). *Path of the Kabbalah.* New York: Paragon House.

Schneerson, M.M., (1995). *Toward a Meaningful Life,* adapted by S. Jacobson. New York: William Morrow and Company Inc.

Wolfensberger, W. (1983). Social Role Valorization: A Proposed New Term for the Principle of Normalization. *Mental Retardation,* 21, 234-239.

Wolfensberger, W. (1988). Common Assets of Mentally Retarded People that are Commonly Not Acknowledged. *Mental Retardation,* 26, 63-70.

A Perspective on the Work of Wolf Wolfensberger

J. Eric Pridmore, MDiv

INTRODUCTION

It has been my experience that many scholars and activists in the disability community take for granted the relationship between religion and disability. While there is much discussion about economic, political, legal, educational, and familial aspects of disability, little attention is paid to the role of religion. Religious attitudes, beliefs, and practices play a significant role in almost every social and cultural context. This point is particularly true for the study of disability. Wolf Wolfensberger genuinely understands this point. For him, a discussion of disability absent a religious component is by definition incomplete. Wolfensberger understands the power of religion to incorporate and exclude individuals. He understands that religious communities provide their members with a way of understanding the larger social world. Thus, Wolfensberger argues, when we exclude mentally retarded individuals from our religious education or worship, we implicitly consent to their overall marginalization in society. Wolfensberger calls the Christian church in particular to fulfill its role in providing a caring, enabling community of support. He understands how important the Christian church's role is in revealing the human worth and dignity of mentally retarded persons. In short, he comprehends the meaningful connections between religion and disability.

In this brief essay, I will examine several of Professor Wolfensberger's articles and presentations. I will begin by looking at how his work has been

J. Eric Pridmore is a PhD Candidate, Drew University, 53 Summerfield Road, Belvidere, NJ 07823 (E-mail: jpridmor@webspan.net).

[Haworth co-indexing entry note]: "A Perspective on the Work of Wolf Wolfensberger." Pridmore, J. Eric. Co-published simultaneously in *Journal of Religion, Disability & Health* (The Haworth Pastoral Press, an imprint of The Haworth Press, Inc.) Vol. 4, No. 2/3, 2001, pp. 139-144; and: *The Theological Voice of Wolf Wolfensberger* (ed: William C. Gaventa, and David L. Coulter) The Haworth Pastoral Press, an imprint of The Haworth Press, Inc., 2001, pp. 139-144. Single or multiple copies of this article are available for a fee from The Haworth Document Delivery Service [1-800-342-9678, 9:00 a.m. - 5:00 p.m. (EST). E-mail address: getinfo@haworthpressinc.com].

helpful to the discussion on religion and disability. I will then offer a critique of his work and examine some potential problems. Finally, I will draw together some general conclusions and insights from the work of Wolfensberger.

IMPORTANT INSIGHTS FROM WOLFENSBERGER

Wolfensberger offers many insightful points in his writing on Christianity and disability. My intention is simply to highlight those points that are from my perspective most helpful. First, it is important to note Wolfensberger's almost exclusive focus on mental retardation and individuals with mental retardation. He brings out the central issues and values encompassing mental retardation and those with this disability. I highlight this obvious point because too often in the disability community we use the terms "disability" and "disabled" to refer to "physical disability" and "physically disabled." Too often people with mental and cognitive disabilities are either ignored or simply forgotten. Wolfensberger reminds us that mental retardation must be a part of the disability discussion. This is true for both the church and the social community at large.

What Wolfensberger and those with cognitive disabilities bring to the discussion is the notion that disability is not something that can be "fixed" with training and adaptive equipment. Disability, both physical and mental, is part of the human condition. Ramps, elevators, dog guides, T.T.D.'s, and other such adaptive tools will, in the long run, fail to bring about equality or justice for people with disabilities if we continue to view disability as an abnormality to be corrected. These tools are important but Wolfensberger, by focusing as he does on cognitive disability, calls attention to the notion that disabilities do not necessarily need correcting. As Wolfensberger puts it, Christian persons with mental retardation speak prophetic words. They speak with inspiration and with courage not in spite of their disability but with and because of their disability. Individuals with mental and physical disabilities are not to be fixed. Rather, they are to be included in the Christian faith community and valued for who they are and the gifts they bring.

The second point I would highlight in Wolfensberger's writing is his conception of religious colonization. Wolfensberger writes, "There must be less glorification of the now almost technological-mechanistic religious education of the handicapped by people who see themselves as in possession of the spiritual goods. . . 'We' must 'reach the retarded'. . . Not 'they reach us,' but 'we reach them.' " Wolfensberger perceives the religious education of persons with disabilities to be virtually the same as the religious colonization by Christians of other continents in the seventeenth and eighteenth centuries. By valuing this type of religious colonization, the church implicitly places people with mental disabilities in an inferior position and segregates them out of the mainstream life of the church. Wolfensberger contends and I would agree that religious education is important and has its place in the life of the religious community. However, when religious education becomes the goal as opposed to the means it crosses over into religious colonization. Wolfensberger's point is that Christian community must be a shared event with the disabled and the able-bodied reaching out to one another in Christian communality.

Moreover, Wolfensberger goes a step further with regard to his conception of religious colonization and segregation by framing it as a moral issue. He writes, "In fact, one may ask further whether there is not an unconscious immorality in most . . . forms of religious education and religious participation that are segregated. There might be hypocrisy in such segregated activities in that religious education is used as yet another endorsement of societal rejection of its unwanted or low-valued members." Wolfensberger challenges the church to see the exclusion of disabled people from mainstream church activities as a moral issue. He also calls the Christian church to make a moral stand against the oppression of people with disabilities in US society. The segregation and colonization of the mentally and physically disabled is a point that must be dealt with seriously. We cannot expect equality and justice in civil society until we can model this behavior in our religious communities. Wolfensberger makes this point clear.

A third major point which should be highlighted in Wolfensberger's writing is his discussion of the treatment of devalued people. In particular, he delineates three primary ways in which devalued individuals are "distantiated," or marginalized. I am not convinced that these are the *only* ways that marginalization takes shape. Nevertheless, I believe Wolfensberger has identified three distinct forms of marginalization. First, according to Wolfensberger, devalued persons can be distantiated or marginalized by physically destroying them. A prime example of this is the systematic killing of people with disabilities in Nazi Germany. As Wolfensberger writes, "This is the ultimate distantiation, the 'final solution.' "

A second approach to marginalizing devalued persons is by creating physical distance by removing the devalued group or by removing one's own group. Wolfensberger points out that social power plays a definite role here in determining who is physically located. As can be seen in the growing suburban sprawl of United States cities, the dominant group will usually remove itself from the devalued and powerless groups. As the devalued begin to move into areas where the dominant group is in the majority, the dominant group begins to relocate. Social scientists have described this as "white flight." Another example of this type of marginalization would be the institutionalization of mentally and physically disabled persons for non-medical reasons.

Wolfensberger describes the third approach to marginalization as the creation of social distance by objectification. According to Wolfensberger, this third approach occurs when physical removal is not possible and when sanctions and morals prevent physical annihilation. Objectification occurs when devalued persons are treated as though they were not really human beings but merely an object. Often times, able-bodied people will go to great lengths to avoid any interaction or contact with a disabled person. When such interaction or contact is unavoidable, the able-bodied individual will not speak directly to the disabled person but to those around her or him. I have personally noticed this type of objectification while dining out with my spouse. On such occasions the server will frequently direct questions about me or my needs to my spouse. This type of behavior is perhaps the most common approach to marginalization.

The purpose of Wolfensberger in this discussion of social marginalization is to call the Christian community into action. According to Wolfensberger, the church has the ability and the responsibility to condemn such social distantiation in whatever form it takes. Moreover, the church has the obligation of exhibiting inclusive behavior by incorporating the mentally and physically disabled into religious education and shared worship.

A CRITIQUE OF WOLFENSBERGER

As I have indicated above, Wolfensberger offers many helpful and insightful points regarding the relationship between the mentally disabled and the Christian church. However, there are several points at which I must disagree with Wolfensberger. I will presently deal with only two of these points.

First, in his discussion of Christian communality, Wolfensberger accuses many Christian pastors of being overly concerned about membership numbers. He writes:

> After all, at least in part for the sake of numbers, Christians condone militarism, war, violence, sexual sins, homosexual behavior, abortion, "euthanasia," and religious services based on Mickey Mouse, Peanuts, and clown themes that open the door to dangerous influences from a media-possessed non-Christian pop culture–one often viewed by contemporary Christians as superior to historical Christian culture.

My initial response to this piece of Wolfensberger's writing is where is the evidence? What data or research exists that in some way proves Wolfensberger's claim? He seems to be arguing not just against large memberships, but also against a great number of other sins within the contemporary church. I find nothing in his writing that substantiates any of his claims against the contemporary church. Moreover, in the research I have done on euthanasia, I have found no evidence to suggest that any US Christian groups support the practice of euthanasia, or, for that matter, violence of any kind. Neither have I found a connection between large-membership churches and support of euthanasia. I contend that such baseless rhetoric by Wolfensberger does not aid his larger argument nor does it help to include people with disabilities into the church.

My second critique of Wolfensberger also refers back to the above quotation. Wolfensberger seems to be arguing that Christian communality compels the church to be loving, supportive, and inclusive of people with mental and physical disabilities. However, within the very same article he condemns homosexuality as "unChristian" and compares it to war, violence, sexual sins, and euthanasia. I do not understand how he can make the argument that the lack of Christian communality is the "central obstacle to proper relationships with needy members" while at the same time harshly excluding a statistically large group desperately in need of the church's ministry. In short, I find his arguments regarding Christian communality completely insincere and harmful to the cause of people with disabilities.

What Wolfensberger appears to be missing is the fact that disability is a socially-constructed category. That is to say, there is no one universal, cross-cultural understanding of what it means to be disabled. Different cultures and different historical eras view disability in dramatically different ways. A facial scar may be mark of the divine in one culture while that very same scar may be a shameful disfigurement in another culture. Likewise, the categories of race, class, gender, and sexual orientation are all culturally-dependent. There is no one universal, cross-cultural understanding of race, class, gender, or sexual orientation. Therefore, if one is going to argue, as I believe Wolfensberger does, that the church and society as a whole should view disabled people as equal and normal human actors, one must also argue that people of any race, class, gender, and sexual orientation are equal and normal human actors. It seems to me that the disabled will never gain complete equality and justice in the church or elsewhere as long as we are willing to aid in the excluding of other "abnormal" individuals.

CONCLUSION

Despite my criticisms, I believe that Wolfensberger offers some unique and compelling insights. His challenge to the Christian church is strong and poignant. His defense of mentally retarded individuals is sound and inspiring. My hope is that more scholars like Wolfensberger will begin to incorporate religious attitudes, beliefs, and practices into their work on disability. This type of discussion and debate is terribly lacking in the disability community.

Finally, I could not agree more with Wolfensberger when he argues that the church should be leading the way in responding to the needs and desires of people with disabilities. Oppression in the United States will not end until religious communities respond to the prophets' call for justice, equality, and social and cultural inclusion. All of us need to hear the prophetic voices described by Wolfensberger.

BOOK REVIEW

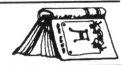

A GUIDELINE ON PROTECTING THE HEALTH AND LIVES OF PA-
TIENTS IN HOSPITALS, ESPECIALLY IF THE PATIENT IS A MEMBER
OF A SOCIETALLY DEVALUED CLASS. Wolfensberger, Wolf. *Syracuse,
NY, self-published, 1992.*

This modest 80-page booklet (only slightly longer than its title) is "a set of
guidelines" to help defend and protect the well-being, "even the life" of a
patient under hospital care. Wolfensberger first defines the problem, as he
sees it, of the dangers inherent in hospitalization and the disproportionate
risks incurred by certain types of patients, "especially where the patient is a
member of a group or class that is societally disadvantaged, or generally held
in low esteem" (page 2). He then offers a variety of practical ways for
concerned persons to protect patients during hospitalization by acting as what
he calls "guardians." The last section discusses problems, issues and concerns that may arise in implementing the program he describes.

To address first the strengths, as "a set of guidelines" this book develops
admirably the concept of "guardians" to safeguard and support at-risk hospital patients, preferably around the clock in shifts. Mr. Wolfensberger apparently has had extensive bedside experience in doing just that, and the guidelines are generally excellent, practical, measured and wise. Families of
vulnerable patients, churches and caring communities, and "circles of
friends" for persons with disabilities can find here an innovative and work-
able, tested manner to support their loved ones through hospitalizations.

What makes the book more complex to review, however, is its sub-text of
concerns for "members of societally devalued classes." The author's creden-

[Haworth co-indexing entry note]: "Book Review." Tittle, Kenneth M. Co-published simultaneously in
Journal of Religion, Disability & Health (The Haworth Pastoral Press, an imprint of The Haworth Press,
Inc.) Vol. 4, No. 2/3, 2001, pp. 145-147; and: *The Theological Voice of Wolf Wolfensberger* (ed: William C.
Gaventa, and David L. Coulter) The Haworth Pastoral Press, an imprint of The Haworth Press, Inc., 2001,
pp. 145-147. Single or multiple copies of this article are available for a fee from The Haworth Document
Delivery Service [1-800-342-9678, 9:00 a.m. - 5:00 p.m. (EST). E-mail address: getinfo@haworthpress
inc.com].

tials to address these topics are not defined. The title page identifies Wolfensberger as Professor, Syracuse University School of Education, and Director, Training Institute for Human Service Planning, Leadership & Change Agentry[sic]. However, his premise is clear as we learn that this book is expanded from an appendix to his book, *The New Genocide of Handicapped and Afflicted People* (Wolfensberger, 1987, second edition 1992).

Wolfensberger provides an interesting analysis of the factors detrimental to good patient care in today's hospitals and of the possibilities and obstacles for improvement. It would be hard for any reasonably informed observer to quarrel with his basic conclusions: (1) Modern acute care hospitals are complex, dangerous places with many possibilities for harming the patients they are meant to serve; (2) The sicker you are, the more danger there is; and (3) certain classes of patients (including the poor, the chronically or terminally ill patient, the mentally or psychiatrically or seriously physically disabled patient, substance abusers, and the obnoxious, among others) are disproportionately at risk for sub-optimal care.

We could argue that these problems are to a degree inevitable realities of modern acute care hospitalization administered by sinners. The "guardian" support system Wolfensberger advocates as "autonomous and corrective" could be valuable for any seriously ill hospitalized patient, and complementary to the professional hospital workers.

However, he goes considerably beyond that. He suggests without documentation that "modern hospital medicine can be said to be in a state of implosion (i.e., a form of collapse) from its own complexity." That would be a credible assertion if it referred to the skyrocketing costs of modern hospital care, but he clearly is implying a dangerous escalation in dangers to the patient, "poorer health outcomes," something the data do not so well support.

He also propagates the unfortunate and widespread "guinea pig" misconception that teaching hospitals are inherently more dangerous because less experienced students and residents participate heavily in the patient's care. There are hassles and disadvantages for teaching hospital patients, but inferior care is not inherently one of them. With histories and physicals being done two and three and more times, multiple specialty consultations, layers of oversight, outstanding senior physicians, good nursing, and all the trainees competing fiercely to demonstrate their competence and to avoid being shown up by those above them, quality of care is often outstanding.

Of greater concern are darkly menacing but undocumented assertions that appear frequently. For example, "Once the decision has been made not to institute special efforts to keep a patient alive, it is then also very common for medical personnel to arrange for death to occur while the family is not present" (page 7). "In recent years there has also been a dramatic rise in human service personnel quite consciously undertaking to kill patients whom they loathed" (page 10). "There have been an increasing number of so-called 'mercy killings' in hospitals and usually they have been quite deliberate" (page 10). Also for Wolfensberger, feeding tubes are simply destructive ways for the nursing staff to shirk responsibilities, interventions that put the patient on the "slippery slope to death," rather than highly successful responses to the malnutrition that was rampant in the old-fashioned hospitals whose passing Wolfensberger laments.

Given the polemical tone and sinister implications of the opening section, I found the middle section, the "nuts and bolts" of the guardian program, to be unexpectedly and refreshingly balanced and fair. I was particularly pleasantly surprised to find him emphasizing the importance for guardians (and their patients) of healthy, positive, non-adversarial relationships with staff and providers, a point he then further underscores in the closing section discussing problems and issues in implementation.

These are trying times in acute care medicine. Increasingly costly and technical methods for extending severely ill patients' lives are available, but their full implementation is opposed by societal fiscal considerations on the one hand and advocates of more humane and accepting treatment of death and dying on the other. (A phenomenal part of our health care resources are expended in the last four weeks of patients' lives, and much of that is not to attain more comfort, peace and quality of life, but rather to buy minutes and hours of sustained metabolism.) Christians' belief in the inherent value of each human life are in tension with a secular society obsessed with "worth" and productivity and status, including the extreme manifestations of the "right to die" and mercy killing for those whose lives are deemed "not worth living." It is a situation rife for sinful exploitation, both from greed and from prejudices.

Persons with disabilities, among others, are rightly concerned. The society as a whole has yet to comprehend the gravity of the situation. Unfortunately, Wolfensberger, who is deeply ambivalent about end of life technology and as well as about allowing patients to die ("death talking"), may well have muddled rather than advanced this crucial national dialogue with his genocide allusions and poorly argued assertions. Nevertheless, his excellent guidelines for guardians can stand for themselves, and are a challenge to us all to get involved at the human level.

Kenneth M. Tittle, MD
Mariposa Ministry
Calexico, CA

WOLF WOLFENSBERGER RESPONDS

Response to the Responders

Wolf Wolfensberger, PhD

My family was a mixture of Jews, Protestants and Catholics, almost all of them nonpracticing, with me being the only member in generations who was a "practicing" believer from infancy. However, I do not recall ever being taught that one's faith, reason, scholarly learning, and occupational functioning should be a coherent whole. I had to learn this bit by bit on my own, but then tried to help others who had also never been taught this to strive for the same goal.

It would be useful for readers of my various publications to keep in mind for whom they were intended, and what their purposes were; some of the reviewers might have taken more note of this. Aside from the short book that was reviewed, all the articles started out as speeches; all were for audiences presumed to be Christian, or interested in Christian perspectives; all were to audiences concerned with mentally retarded people, or else I would have said more about other devalued conditions and classes–as I actually did in other contexts; three of the speeches were prepared for primarily mixed Christian audiences, and four for Catholic ones; the "How We Carry the Ministry . . ." and "The Most Urgent Issues . . ." articles were very abbreviated summaries of much longer talks, which created many problems in transmitting the message.

[Haworth co-indexing entry note]: "Response to the Responders." Wolfensberger, Wolf. Co-published simultaneously in *Journal of Religion, Disability & Health* (The Haworth Pastoral Press, an imprint of The Haworth Press, Inc.) Vol. 4, No. 2/3, 2001, pp. 149-157; and: *The Theological Voice of Wolf Wolfensberger* (ed: William C. Gaventa, and David L. Coulter) The Haworth Pastoral Press, an imprint of The Haworth Press, Inc., 2001, pp. 149-157. Single or multiple copies of this article are available for a fee from The Haworth Document Delivery Service [1-800-342-9678, 9:00 a.m. - 5:00 p.m. (EST). E-mail address: getinfo@haworthpressinc.com].

149

Also, in the 1970s, I was responding to the fact that denominations were not accepting of impaired people because society, still stamped by the ideology of social Darwinism, was not accepting them. In other words, church practice was stamped by the world. There were some ministries directed specifically to groups made up entirely of retarded persons, but these were rare. Mostly, there were Protestant ministers, and a smaller number of Catholic priests, who served in institutions; and there were a handful of Catholic priests who had what amounted to special empires (buildings, independent funding sources, great autonomy, etc.) of ministry to retarded persons which they guarded jealously. I remember that when I began teaching to Christian audiences that retarded people belonged in the church congregations, I was and felt alone. I could not even find post-medieval treatises that explicated a Christian perspective on this, and my 1979 article reflected a desperate struggle to identify relevant rationales. I also remember making, at least initially, little impact on the listeners with my message of integrating retarded people into generic congregations and religious services. L'Arche was a partial exception; while it congregated retarded persons, it at least actively recruited nonretarded people to come to them not only in service but in living together, in sociability, and in religious participation.

As to the specific responders, Schurter seems to have understood best what I intended to convey, though he makes me squirm (and also snicker a bit about my wretched sinfulness) by mentioning Jeremiah, Hosea, Amos, John the Baptizer and Wolfensberger in virtually the same breath. I can only hope they were even bigger sinners than I. I am also thankful to him for pointing out how the five elements that I posited as making for "the good life" for retarded persons are all tied together by the theme of communality. I also agree with him that the message of Christian communality has hardly been heard, or accepted, by most Christians. Many do teach the new secular religion of "inclusion," but not of Christian communality; thereby, they once again let the world dictate to them what form Christianity should take, rather than Christianity demonstrating to the world what Christianity is supposed to be like.

Bersani's introduction was rather clever–almost too much so–but it may shed further light on me to reveal that when I came to Syracuse University in 1973, and they asked me what I wanted to name "my thing," I took a deep breath and blurted out "Training Institute for Human Service Planning, Leadership and Change Agentry," fully expecting my listeners to convulse in laughter. No one laughed, so I thought to myself, "ok, then that is what you'll get."

Next, I will explain two things that are relevant to several responses. First, a crucially important spiritual discipline is to identify idols. Among their characteristics is that (a) they make extravagant promises, (b) once established, they demand that their worshippers bring human sacrifices (which these days, are rarely recognized as such, abortion being a striking example), and (c) they eventually betray their worshippers. This will have a bearing on several of my more specific responses. Secondly, when a new practice or trend comes along, one should search to know whether it springs from godly or ungodly sources. If it springs from ungodly ones, one should (a) deeply distrust it, and (b) search to know what bad purposes it may be serving or what harm it generates. If the new development is an outright ideology, one should try to scrutinize it especially hard in order to identify its underlying– and usually unexplicated–"religion," and whether it is an idolatry. Of course, one must not be fooled by the fact that the development does some good, because even the greatest evil comes with some benefits.

Building on the two disciplines mentioned above, it is relevant to several responses that one of the leading secular religions today is radical individualism, and derived from it, one of the leading religions in human services is an intertwined web of constructs of self-determination, self-advocacy, "choice," and "empowerment." These do not come from God or friends of God, but from the idolatry of the human, and specifically the individual human (in contrast to the idolatry of the human collectivity that marked Marxism). Relevant countervailing Christian ideals are obedience; submission and mutual submission; interdependence; and surrender of power. Several of these might possibly take the forms of surrender of options, voluntary poverty, or being with and becoming like the lowly. Power specifically is allied to material force, hence material violence, while in contrast, Christianity (I believe) calls for nonviolence. As John Howard Yoder (e.g., 1972) taught, there really *is* a "politics of Jesus," but so few Christians seem to know, understand or believe it, or act even modestly in accord with it; in fact, most Americans at least do not understand what politics is. Among the many human sacrifices of the idol of individualism is the abandonment of people of impaired (or even absent) mental competency to their own "choices," self-advocacy and self-determination. (The very term "choice" has become popular because of its legitimization of the human sacrifice of the unborn.) Among the betrayals of this idol of modernism is that it is giving us a decadent, decommunitizing, decommunitized, nonviable and collapsing culture.

Also, at least portions of several responses brought out that when one is exposed to a high-level view (be it a religious, philosophical, cultural, or even other secular position or theory) that is different from one's own, one is not only likely to disagree, but one may not even understand it, and therefore, one will not be able to explain it accurately to others. I believe that this was a major problem with certain points of critique that needed nuance, nuance and more nuance. Marc Gold (may he rest in peace) wrote a book entitled, *Did I Say That?* (1980). I could write not just one such book, but a whole series of them, because people constantly attribute sayings or positions to me that were never mine.

Here are some corrections to various mistaken presentations of my writings and views by one or more responders. I have never believed or stated that "all change is bad," or that "progress should be stopped" (or even can be); I certainly have not "denied knowledge and progress," nor had much fear of the unknown (I do fear some of what we know, and so should everyone else); I see many of the contemporary problems of science and technology as being largely derivative of the materialized religion of modernism, and as becoming problems precisely because they are cut loose from the control of valid moral worldviews and principles; I do not see them as free-standing problems. Nor did I mean to convey that people are turning to Eastern religions *primarily* because science and technology have failed; they do so for mostly other reasons, including that materialism is failing, but they detest Christianity.

Several responders–much like almost everybody else–seem enamored of intellectuality, science, technology and medicine. This raises the question whether one reads the developments of one's time with a spiritual eye, or a worldly (these days, materialized) eye. These days, technological developments are virtually never read with a spiritualized eye, even by people who are prepared to read many other developments with a bit more spiritualization. And if one takes technology into one's soul, one will come to love technological developments very uncritically. For instance, one may end up believing things such as that one can have nuclear power without getting nuclear weapons, or even without nuclear pollution. The fact that citizens loyal to modernism (as most people now are) cannot see even its sinister technological side reminds me of the Germans who, even days before Germany's surrender in 1945, still believed in victory by their idol–some continued to believe it even after the surrender, and some of that very generation are still Nazis to this day.

What is amazing is that in an age where even non-believers have become more prepared to see beyond the surface of things (as evidenced in the analysis of systems, in constructivism, even in psychotherapy), so many people of religious faith do not want to start looking beyond the surface of these or many other things. Of course, people are particularly unprepared to be critical toward their idols, and science and technology is one of the major idols of our age. However, one need not rely on Wolfensberger's analysis or intuition on these things, since in recent decades, a good number of eminent people from a wide range of both religious and secular backgrounds have published trenchant critiques of these, and intellectuals should be aware of what at least some of the points of criticism are. It is also painful that some of this even needs to be mentioned in the face of realities such as are daily in the news (e.g., the explosion of Littleton-type, and people running murderously amok, phenomena), and in face of problems such as the Y2K computer snafu–this one being an example of a problem that was utterly predictable, but nonetheless designed by the world's smartest people who now control much of our lives, and which may "bomb" parts of the Third World into a state where, for the foreseeable future, they will reap the worst of modernism with none of its benefits.

I will, however, clarify my above disavowals by confessing that I had fervently hoped that all rich people's computers (poor people rarely have any) would fail on 1 January 2000, so that they would not be able to chat with their therapists or support group members thousands of miles away, and would start smelling the rancid bacon. Oh Lord, how long? When will the upper crust have their ivories taken away (Amos 6:4) so that they will have to write their texts about naive Luddites with goose quills?

Several readers seem exercised (not exorcised but exercised) over the fact that I have occasionally used the terms "Satan" and "satanic" (the divinity schools and theology departments have done a thorough job here!). However, insofar as Satan is mentioned at least 54 times in scripture (including 19 times in the Jewish books), and at least 12 of these times by Christ (to say nothing of Beelzebub, the devil, or devils being mentioned at least 106 other times, some also by Christ), I need hardly feel ashamed, being in such good company–much better than the company of overeducated theologians. What I do believe is that there are fallen angels in opposition to God, and that they are no idle bystanders in the moral realm. However, where formerly I may have said "satanic," I would probably say "demonic" today.

To clarify another and related issue that seemed on the minds of several readers: affliction, disease, aging, stupidity, insanity, suffering, imperfection–even such things as forgetting, and functioning unconsciously–I believe to be results and manifestations of the human fall from the originally created condition first of human nature, and secondly of the material universe. Humans were not meant to be thusly imperfect and beset, nor will they be when on the day known but to God, all things (theologians, take note: except the fallen angels and God-hating humans) are restored once again to their pre-fallen condition.

I believe that it is relevant to both Friedman's and Pridmore's comments to distinguish that there are extremely strong empirical rationales for acceptance and integration of impaired people; there are also very clear supra-empirical rationales from a variety of religious/philosophical perspectives; and then there are explicitly Christian rationales. As to the issue of Christian communality specifically, the point was not that handicapped people belonging to any group (even an atheistic one) is good, but that in my opinion, Christianity specifically was meant to be quintessentially communal, and that if Christian congregations do not manage to be communal, or do not even believe that they ought to be, then we cannot expect them to be communal toward impaired and dependent persons. Friedman is correct that I should have said more about at least the genuinely communal family as a model for other communalities, but Christianity teaches that one's Christian faith may divide one from one's family, and that then, fellow believers–at least if they properly practice their faith–become "brother, sister and mother" (Matthew 12:50; Mark 3:34-35; see also Matthew 19:29, Luke 18:29) to one. Indeed, if a person from a traditional Jewish or Islamic family should become a Christian, then the person could expect to be shunned by his/her family (in Islam, even killed), and would be in a bad situation if the Christian community did not become his/her new family.

I detect more than a whiff of political correctness in some of Pridmore's comments (but also a whiff of a whiff in Bersani's), which is why those of us with intellectual gifts and high education need to spend much time around lowly, uneducated and unintelligent people.

In regard to Pridmore, first, some human conditions are variations more than abnormalities, but some are violations of, or deviations from, or failures of, what one might call entelechy, i.e., humans were not meant by God or nature to have these conditions–not even within the era of the Fall. A cow with three or five legs is a failure of entelechy, as is a person without ears, without a cerebrum, or with four eyes. These are not merely statistical anomalies but entelechic ones. Nor is there anything wrong with attempts to correct or compensate for such or other abnormalities, e.g., with efforts to strengthen feeble hands, and to straighten or steady "tottering knees" (Isaiah 35:3)–as long as such efforts do not spring from a conditionality mentality, i.e., a mentality that interprets the person without ears or with four eyes as non-human, as a non-person, as not of equal value with the entelechally perfect one, or as not a suitable member of one's congregation (provided the person truly wants to be a member). (If there were no such words as entelechic, and entelechally, there are now, and should have been before now.)

Secondly, I did not condemn homosexuality (though I see it as a failure of entelechy, or as a body-mind incoherency, and like any serious incoherency no cause for celebration). I did say that "homosexual behavior" (by which I meant homosexual acts) is to be no more condoned by Christian bodies than war, violence, other sexual sins, Mickey Mouse religious services, etc. However, there have always been many homosexual people who love and obey God, even are saintly, and who do not approve of, or engage in, homosexual acts.

Thirdly, everyone needs to understand that if one were to embrace a Christianized version of the kind of extreme cultural relativism that is currently the craze in the anti-Christian, indeed anti-theistic, world of secular politically correct constructionism that rather peculiarly has substituted "multiculturalism" and "diversity" for morality, or even for religion, then this would imply two things, among others (including that the world is once again dictating what Christianity should be and believe). (a) There could be no such thing as natural law, as posited in most strands of Christianity, by some other religions, and even rather illogically by some atheists. (b) One would have to deny (as constructionists generally do) that there is anything genetically "hard-wired" in the human, as if one of the burdens of the Fall were not the demonic little joke (or perhaps an arty conceit) that we have animal bodies; surely, we did not have monkey bodies in Paradise!

Fourthly, war, violence in law enforcement, violence in self-defense, violence in disciplining persons, and capital punishment have been defended by almost all Christian churches; various forms of euthanasia have been explicitly endorsed by several Christian denominations; and abortion (at least under certain circumstances) has been legitimized by almost all. If one does not believe this, one must do more "research." Even a majority of "pro-life" people have been revealed (by "research") to approve of abortion as a response to prenatal diagnoses of anomalies, conception from rape or incest, or appreciable danger to the health or life of the mother–all very "practical" positions!

Specifically to Friedman's response, readers might be left with the mistaken impression that hers reflects a Jewish perspective. This is why it would have been much clearer and more useful if she had explicated which of the Christian positions I presented are, or are not, shared by Judaism generally; which are shared only by Hasidic (or at least orthodox) Judaism; and which are, or are not, shared by Friedman for her own personal reasons. For instance, the Jewish Bible itself emphatically and repeatedly teaches that turning away from God makes one stupid, by which it usually means in a wisdom sense (i.e., making one what the Greeks called amathic or foolish) which, however, can easily be shown to potentially also lead to stupidity in the natural sense; and that vice versa, the simple can become wise by taking in, and trusting, the word of God. On the role of prophecy specifically, a rabbinic adage popular since the second century AD has been: "From the fall of the second temple, prophecy was taken from the prophets (i.e., those who ordinarily practiced it) and given to fools and infants." (Golda Meir cited this proverb on her 74th birthday.) Rabbi Kushner, cited by Friedman, has made a name for himself by questioning the omnipotence of God ("when bad things happen to good people"), which is surely a scandal to orthodox Jewish teaching, and probably even to most conservative Jews, thus revealing that one must nuance what a Jewish position is.

My monograph, *A Guideline on Protecting the Health & Lives of Patients in Hospitals, Especially if the Patient Is a Member of a Societally Devalued Class*, was a secular publication for ordinary people. In response to Tittle's skepticism about some of the warnings in it, there does indeed exist mountainous evidence both as to the dangerousness of all medical care, the dangerousness of hospitals specifically, and the danger to societally devalued people from the medical system. Not only the medical journals, but the generic news media have been reporting things such as that in hospitals, poor post-operative nutrition is a big contributor to post-operative death; that annually, between 1.3-2.0 million Americans have harm done to them in/by hospitals; that there is an average of one drug error per hospital patient per day, and that in an average large hospital, 30-60 such errors are committed per hour; that up to 300,000 cases of ill done in hospitals involve negligence; that 100,000 people die from these episodes; that 90,000 die from infections caught in hospitals; and that drug prescription and dispensing errors outside of hospitals are so common that they caused 2.7 million hospital admissions in the US in the early 1980s. We can also read local horror stories about such problems in specific hospitals: waves of errors and deaths, hospital wings shut down because of dangerous ineradicable germs in them, etc. Societally devalued people are hit harder by each and every such problem category. Comparable data are reported from other developed Western countries. Even the mainstream of medicine now admits that hospitals are very dangerous places, which is one reason (other than cost-cutting) why (a) as many operations as possible are now carried out on an outpatient basis, and (b) why hospital stays are made as short as possible. Johns Hopkins only recently reported that outpatient breast surgery results in (a) fewer infections, and (b) more satisfied patients. There exist entire "pediatric hospitals" where virtually all children (mostly impaired ones) are tube-fed as a matter of convenience, and all are expected to die. Documentation on "deathmaking" of devalued people in medical settings, or under medical care outside of medical settings, is now mountainous. Entire journals are devoted to the topic (e.g., the *International Anti-Euthanasia Task Force's Update* is one of the best in this category). Books have been written on secret medical killings (e.g., Beine, 1998, about several countries), mostly of debilitated patients. *The Guidelines* itself points readers to Wolfensberger (1992b) for more details. However, there would be people who would know such things even if they were not documented by research. I, for one, might have been made out a fool or paranoid for claiming such things–as I indeed was before "research" made it official. But such documentation does not belong in a booklet such as *The Guidelines*, nor do I think I should do this work here. (There must be websites with this kind of information!) However, the more one has faith in modern high-tech medicine, the less will one even want to know these facts, and blatant denial thereof actually continues even in circles that are exposed to the documentation.

Relevant both to this issue, and one of Friedman's comments, is that it is not only via medical euthanasia that lowly people are made dead. The scope of abortion (including via search-and-destroy campaigns against impaired babies) is almost beyond comprehension. There is much medical infanticide, there is much deadly violence by families and citizens toward the handicapped, a huge proportion of the mentally handicapped get put on extremely unhealthy prescription mind drugs, and even among relatively healthy retarded persons, extremely few live out their normal life expectancy.

The editors restricted my response to a few pages, so I have to forego further text. However, I believe that this format of debate and analysis is very much what we need because I expect that it will lead to much clarification of thought.

REFERENCES

Beine, K. H. (1998). *Sehen, hören, schweigen: Patiententötungen und active Sterbehilfe*. Freiburg, Germany: Lambertus Verlag.

Gold, M. L. (1980). *Did I say that?: Articles and commentary on the "try another way" system*. Champaign, IL: Research Press.

Wolfensberger, W. (1992a). *A guideline on protecting the health and lives of patients in hospitals, especially if the patient is a member of a societally devalued class*. Syracuse, NY: Training Institute for Human Service Planning, Leadership and Change Agentry (Syracuse University).

Wolfensberger, W. (1992b). *The new genocide of handicapped and afflicted people* (rev. ed.). Syracuse, NY: Training Institute for Human Service Planning, Leadership and Change Agentry (Syracuse University).

Yoder, J. H. (1972). *The politics of Jesus*. Grand Rapids, MI: Wm. B. Eerdmans.

Index

Abductions, of mentally-retarded people, 29-30
Abel, 31
Abortion, 28,80,93,94,101,114, 128,136,142,146-147, 151,152-153
Abuse, of mentally-retarded people, 16-17,27-30
Accullier, 55
Acts 2, 26
Acts 2: 42-47, 116
Acts 3:10, 123
Acts 4, 116
Acts 4:32-35, 111-112
Acts 4:34-35, 121
Acts 7:52, 92
Adulteresses, Christ's relationship with, 61
Advocacy
  citizen, 7,8
  by mentally-retarded people, 4-5,147
  for mentally-retarded people, 82
Alienation
  between God and humanity, 86
  from manual labor, 92-93
  from nature, 93
American Association for the Advancement of Science, 3
American Association of University Professors, 3
American Association on Mental Deficiency (Retardation), 3,4,136-137
  Religion Division of, 33-34,127
American Journal of Mental Deficiency, 7
American Men and Women of Science, 3
American Psychological Association, 3

Amos, 128,146
Amos 6:4, 149
Anabaptist movement, 113-114
Angels, 71,72,77
  fallen, 149
Anglican Church, Task Force on Human Life, 58
Animals
  as caregivers for children, 43-44
  human characteristics of, 39-40
Archbishop of Canterbury, 27
Arche. See L'Arche
Associations for Retarded Citizens/Arc's, 3
Authority, 36,135

Babylon, 35
Bankruptcy, intellectual, 31-33,135-136
Baptism, of mentally-retarded people, 56
Beelzebub, 149
Berrigan, Daniel, 36
Berrigan, Philip, 36
Bersani, Hank, 146,150
Biology, scientific discoveries in, 92
Blatt, Burton, 2
Blessings, as Jewish tradition, 133-134
Body, relationship with the soul, 71-73,76
Body of Christ, 127
  unity of, 88,89
Bonds, social, disruption of, 96
Book review, 155-157
Brahe, Tycho, 42-43
Branding
  physical, of mentally-retarded people, 29

Fabiola, 54,85-86
Fallen nature, of humans, 128,136,149
Family
   versus Christian communality,
     137,150
   law and legal practice related to, 93
Faust, 37
Fear, of the new, 135
Feral children, 43-44
"Feral man," 43
Fertilization, 79-80
Feuerbach, Anselm Ritter von, 46
Fiestas, 25-26,27
Formalization, of social processes, 96
Foucault, Michel, 8
Francis, Saint, 25-26
Francis I, King of France, 42
Frederick the Wise, Duke of Saxony,
   42
Free will, 8,134
Friedman, Sandra, 149,151,152-153
Funeral services, for mentally-retarded
   people, 23

Gender, cultural-dependency of, 143
Genesis 4:14, 31
Genesis 11, 32
Genetic engineering, 93-94
Genetics, 57,92,93
Genocide, 94,95,96-97,101-102,156
Gentling effect, of mentally-retarded
   people, 21-23
George Peabody College for Teachers,
   2
Germ weapons, 93-94
God
   authority of, 36
   mentally-retarded people's
     resistance to,
     74-75,77,79,135
   presence of, 24,27
God's house, 55
Godshuizen, 55
Goethe, Johann Wolfgang, 37,74
Good Friday, 121

Good life, 129,146
Good news, 99-102
Good Samaritan, 61
Group homes, 20,37
*Guidelines on Protecting the Health
   and Lives of Patients. . .*
   (Wolfensberger), 151
   review of, 155-157
Gurus, 93

Habits of the Heart (Bellah), 129
Handicapped people
   early Christians' attitudes toward,
     54
   Nazis' extermination of, 38-39,58
Harmony, paradisial, 88
Hauser, Caspar, 30-31,39
Heaven. *See* Paradise
Hedonism, 93,97,135
"Hessian Wolf Boy," 43
High-school students, 21-23
History, Christian view of, 85-87
Holiness
   of community, 137
   of mentally-retarded people, 79,81
Holocaust, 94,96-97
Homes, sharing of, 90
Homosexuality
   Christians' condonement of,
     114,142,143
   unChristian nature of, 143,150
Hosea, 128,146
Hospices, 54-56,57
Hospital patients, protection of,
   151-152,155-157
Hôtel Dieu, 55
House of Baden, 45,46-47
Hugo, Victor, 42
Human sacrifice, 146-147
Human services
   of Christian churches
     government subsidies for, 119
     historical development of, 54-58
     as ministry, 89-90
     by non-Christians, 118

T - #0554 - 101024 - C0 - 212/152/10 - PB - 9780789013156 - Gloss Lamination